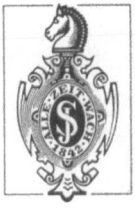

Progress in Pediatric Surgery

Volume 21

Trachea and Lung Surgery in Childhood

Volume Editor
P. Wurnig, Vienna

With 75 Figures

Springer-Verlag
Berlin Heidelberg New York
London Paris Tokyo

Primarius Professor Dr. PETER WURNIG
Chirurgische Abteilung des
Mautner Markhof'schen Kinderspitals
der Stadt Wien
Baumgasse 75, A-1030 Wien

Volumes 1–17 of this series were published by Urban & Schwarzenberg,
Baltimore–Munich

ISBN-13: 978-3-642-71667-6   e-ISBN-13: 978-3-642-71665-2
DOI: 10.1007/978-3-642-71665-2

Library of Congress Cataloging-in-Publication Data. Trachea and lung surgery in childhood.
(Progress in pediatric surgery; v. 21). Includes index. 1. Trachea – Stenosis – Surgery. 2. Trachea
– Surgery. 3. Lungs – Surgery. I. Wurnig, Peter. II. Series. [DNLM: 1. Lung – surgery. 2.
Trachea – surgery. 3. Tracheal Stenosis – in infancy & childhood. W1 PR677KA v. 21 / WF 490
T7588]
RD137.A1P7   vol. 21   [RF516]   617'.98 s   86-31420
ISBN 0-387-17232-7 (U.S.)   [617.533059]

Typesetting and printing: Petersche Druckerei GmbH & Co. Offset KG, Rothenburg ob der Tauber
Bookbinding: Konrad Triltsch, Graphischer Betrieb, D-8700 Würzburg

2123/3130-543210

Preface

With improvements in respirator therapy and intensive care, congenital malformations and various acquired pathologic deformities of the trachea or bronchi are more often observed than used to be the case. For a while it seemed that tracheostomy would be unnecessary, but it has since become quite clear that severe disturbance of the trachea would be the outcome owing to primary or secondary pathologic changes that had not been given adequate consideration previous. These changes can lead to urgent life-threatening episodes or definite mutilation for the rest of the child's life. Tracheal surgery thus represents a new and special challenge for the pediatric surgeon. A solution to these serious problems must be found and merits discussion. Furthermore, it seems worthwhile to review cases of surgical pulmonary diseases, except for the already widely discussed problems of empyemas or bronchiectasis.

P. WURNIG, Vienna

Contents

List of Editors and Contributors

Editors

Angerpointner, T. A., Dr., Kinderchirurgische Klinik im Dr. von Haunerschen Kinderspital der Universität München, Lindwurmstraße 4, D-8000 München 2

Hecker, W. Ch., Prof. Dr., Kinderchirurgische Klinik im Dr. von Haunerschen Kinderspital der Universität München, Lindwurmstraße 4, D-8000 München 2

Rickham, P.P., Prof. Dr. M.D., M.S., F.R.C.S., F.R.C.S.I., F.R.A.C.S., D.C.H., F.A.A.P., Universitätskinderklinik, Chirurgische Abteilung, Steinwiesstraße 75, CH-8032 Zürich

Prévot, J., Prof., Clinique Chirurgical Pédiatrique, Hôpital d'Enfants de Nancy, F-54511 Vandœvre Cedex

Spitz, L., Prof., PhD. FRCS, Nuffield Professor of Pediatric Surgery, Institute of Child Health, University of London, Hospital for Sick Children, Great Ormond Street, 30 Guilford Street, GB-London WC1N 1EH

Stauffer, U. G., Prof. Dr., Universitätskinderklinik, Kinderchirurgische Abteilung, Steinwiesstraße 75, CH-8032 Zürich

Wurnig, P., Prof. Dr., Kinderchirurgische Abteilung des Mautner Markhof'schen Kinderspitals, Baumgasse 75, A-1030 Wien

Contributors

You will find the addresses at the beginning of the respective contribution

Pathophysiology of Subglottic Tracheal Stenosis in Childhood

B. Minnigerode[1] and H. G. Richter[1]

The subglottic space is a region of the airway that is not well defined anatomically, extending in its widest definition from the vocal cord down to the smallest bronchi. In this paper the term is used to mean only as the spatium subglotticum, the space enclosed ventrally and laterally by the elastic cone, which bears the cricoid plate in its posterior wall and which then without a break becomes the cervical trachea at the caudal end of the cricoid cartilage.

There is a variety of causes of stenoses in this segment of the airway, only two particularly problematic types of which will be discussed: (1) *Disturbed embryonic development,* typically giving rise to primary lesions, and (2) *trauma,* which leads mainly to secondary lesions.

1. *Embryonic developmental disturbances* in this area result in so-called hard and soft stenoses of the subglottic space (Minnigerode and Richtering 1969; Minnigerode 1969, 1971). This means a narrowing of the normal shape of the infraglottic conus with a pad-like swelling of the mucosa, reducing the lumen to less than 4 mm in most instances. The basis is probably a metabolic disturbance during the 9th embryonic week, i.e., during the break-off of the physiological epithelial occlusion (Kallius 1897; Minnigerode 1962), which involves all three sections of the larynx. During this developmental stage the epithelium is actually an intermediate layer, a diathelium in the statically and dynamically defined metabolic field between liquid-rich connective tissue and embryonic amniotic fluid. A disturbance of the normal continuous reorganization which typically also takes place in the development of other hollow organs in the human organism (Singer 1933) results in uneven growth of the tissues making up this airway region, an overgrowth of the mesenchymal tissue contrasting with normal growth or hypotrophy of the epithelium. The epithelium is then damaged by the pressure of the mesenchymal pads, and the mesenchymal tissues of both sides may advance and even grow together in an interlocking pattern through the epithelial defects. The kind of stenosis resulting from this depends on whether the maximum of this growth disturbance is more ventrally or more dorsally located, i.e., within the region of the chondrification centre of the cricoid area (Heineken 1952; Walender 1955; Smith and Bain 1965).

Clinically, this kind of stenosis presents as an inspiratory stridor from birth on, initially without obvious impairment of respiration. Impairment of respiration,

---

[1] University Hospital for Otorhinolaryngology, D-4300 Essen, FRG.

Progress in Pediatric Surgery, Vol. 21
Ed. by P. Wurnig
© Springer-Verlag Berlin Heidelberg 1987

which develops typically during the 4th to 6th week after birth, is probably induced at this time by a reduced number of erythrocytes and impaired oxygen transport, and progresses rapidly to the full clinical picture of the subglottic syndrome (Mounier-Kuhn and Gaillard 1962), characterized by dyspnoea of various degrees, voice disturbances (bitonal voice, hoarseness), coughing, expectoration and, frequently, an opisthotonus-like posture effecting a slight enlargement of the subglottic space and consequently easier respiration.

2. *Traumatic stenoses* are the result of an insult to a normal, healthy tissue structure in the subglottic region. Internal injuries are therefore by far the most frequent cause in childhood. Their pathophysiological course may be explained with reference to postintubational stenosis, as an example, although analogous explanations can be given for all other injuries to the internal integument (e.g. foreign bodies, faulty tracheotomy, laryngotracheoscopy).

The triggering cause is frequently tangential tissue damage, which is itself caused even by the inevitable physiological movement of the airway, or by changes in posture, feeding, suction or similar. Two different reactions occur, which proceed in parallel and influence each other to some extent:

1. *Mechanical damage to the surface,* leading rapidly to leucocyte invasion into the subepithelial tissue, perivascular oedema of the connective tissue with maximal enlargement of small veins, a distinct increase in elastic fibres and marked inflammation of the subepithelial tissue in the further course. The result of this is a secondary, circumscribed or more extended, epithelial defect, setting free or even destroying the basal membrane and finally effecting direct damage to the connective tissue.

2. *Irritation of the mucous membrane in the form of a foreign body reaction,* which effects a marked increased in mucus production around the endotracheal tube. The result is a stagnation of secretion in this airway area, associated with massive bacterial contamination, leucocyte invasion into the subepithelial layers, marked enlargement of small veins and perivascular oedema of the connective tissue, which in turn leads to a disturbed blood supply to the excretory ducts. In a phase of high metabolic activity this causes oxygen deficiency of the excretory glands with subsequent autolysis of the glands and extensive inflammation of the surrounding tissue.

The course of these reactions is shown in Figs. 1 and 2.

Remarkably, subepithelial mesenchymal tissues also play a leading role in the origin of traumatic stenoses, and epithelial changes or defects are only secondary lesions. Conspicuous parallels to the pachydermia laryngis diffusa (Virchow 1887) and to the chronic subglottic laryngitis in adults (Minnigerode 1965) can be demonstrated, so that the sequence of inflammatory reactions in the subepithelial connective tissue with thickening of the connective tissue and secondary epithelial lesion seems to be a typical reaction of these airway areas to a stronger, physiologically intolerable mechanical load.

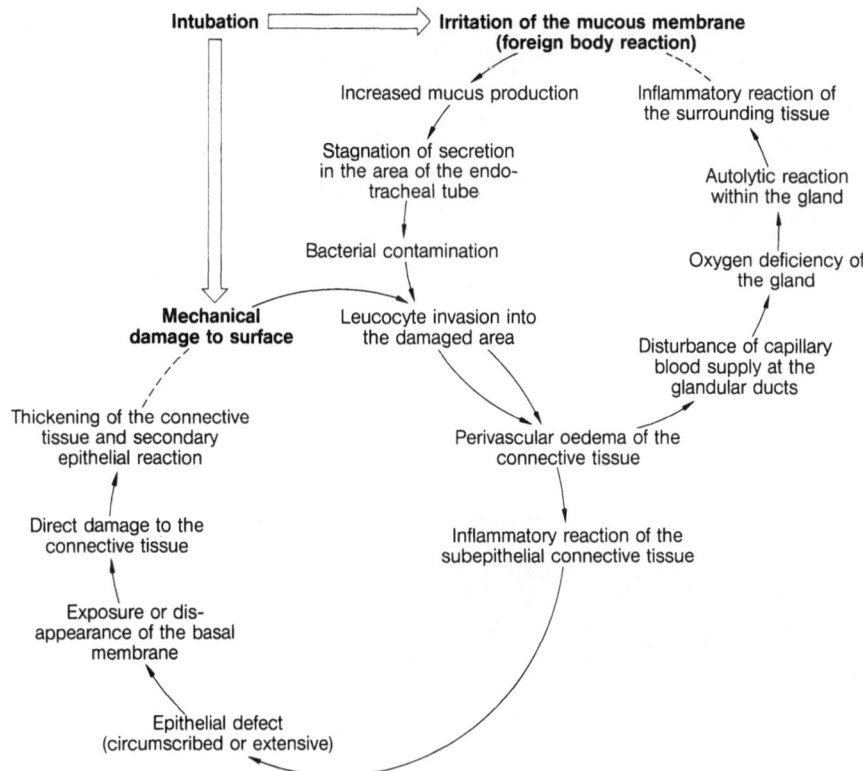

Fig. 1. Schematic of reaction sequence in the origin of traumatic stenoses

If the cause of damage is abolished at this stage the epithelium in the damaged areas regenerates rapidly, whereas the connective tissue reaction regularly continues for a longer time. Therefore, a seemingly normal endoscopic appearance of wall and lumen has no prognostic force with reference to the possible development of a stenosis and its extent.

If, however, the mechanical tissue irritation continues, mucous membrane areas are mostly formed which have grossly impaired ciliary function or are even stripped of the ciliated epithelium. This inevitably leads to an accumulation and deposit of mucous secretion, which in turn maintains a locally confined inflammation because of the inevitable bacterial contamination, preventing regeneration of the ciliated epithelium. All this results in a picture similar to the formerly frequent postendoscopic laryngotracheitis.

In conclusion, particular attention must be devoted to the subepithelial tissues in every kind of treatment of stenoses in this airway region (Meyer 1971; Padovan and Orescovic 1971; Minnigerode and Küpper 1977); the microscopic changes generally exceed the macroscopically recognizable changes in both cranial and caudal directions (Minnigerode et al. 1980).

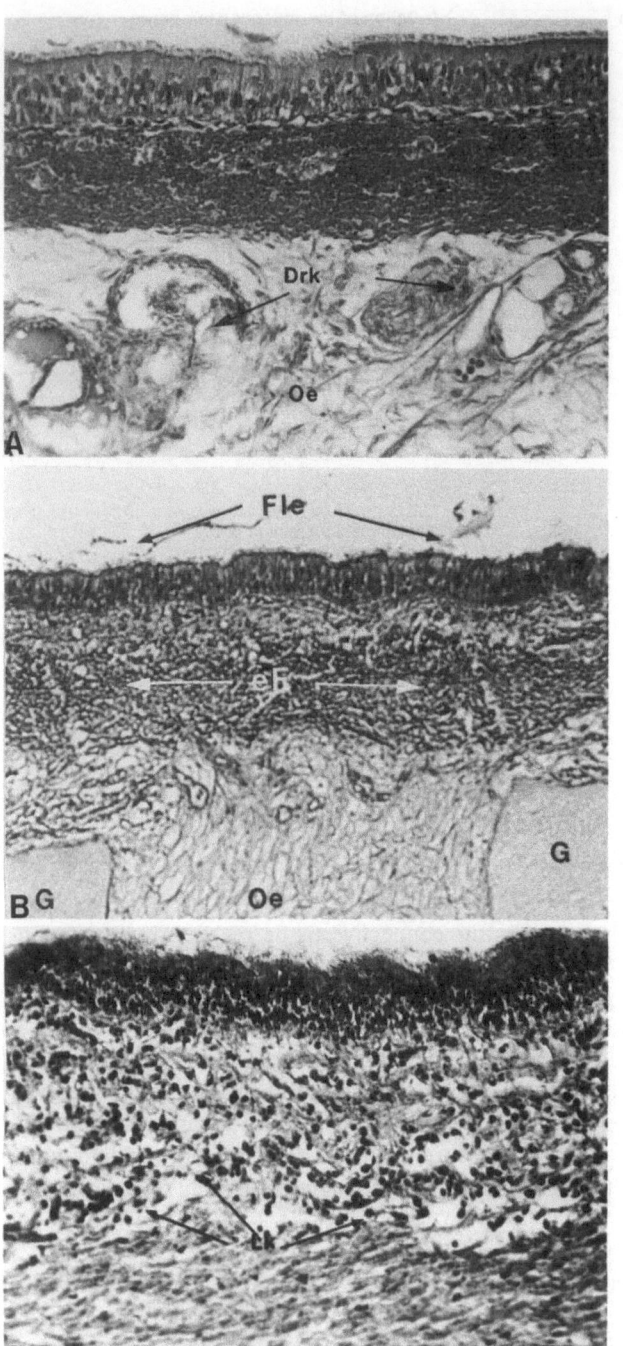

Fig. 2A–F. Histological appearance of the mucous membrane following intubation for 24 h. **A–C** Intact ciliated epithelium *(FLE)*, compact, partly bloated subepithelial elastic fibre zone *(eF)*, marked oedema of the connective tissue *(Oe)*, congested blood vessels *(G)*, leucocyte infiltration *(LK)*. Paraffin sections **A** × 90, **B** × 70, **C** × 100. **D** Scanning electron micrograph of adhering ciliary bunches; × 4000. **E** Scanning electron micrograph of reticulated mucous structures on the ciliated epithelium; × 2000. **F** Scanning electron micrograph of adhering cilia *(Z)*, with massive bacterial contamination *(BK)* of the mucus *(MC)*; × 5200

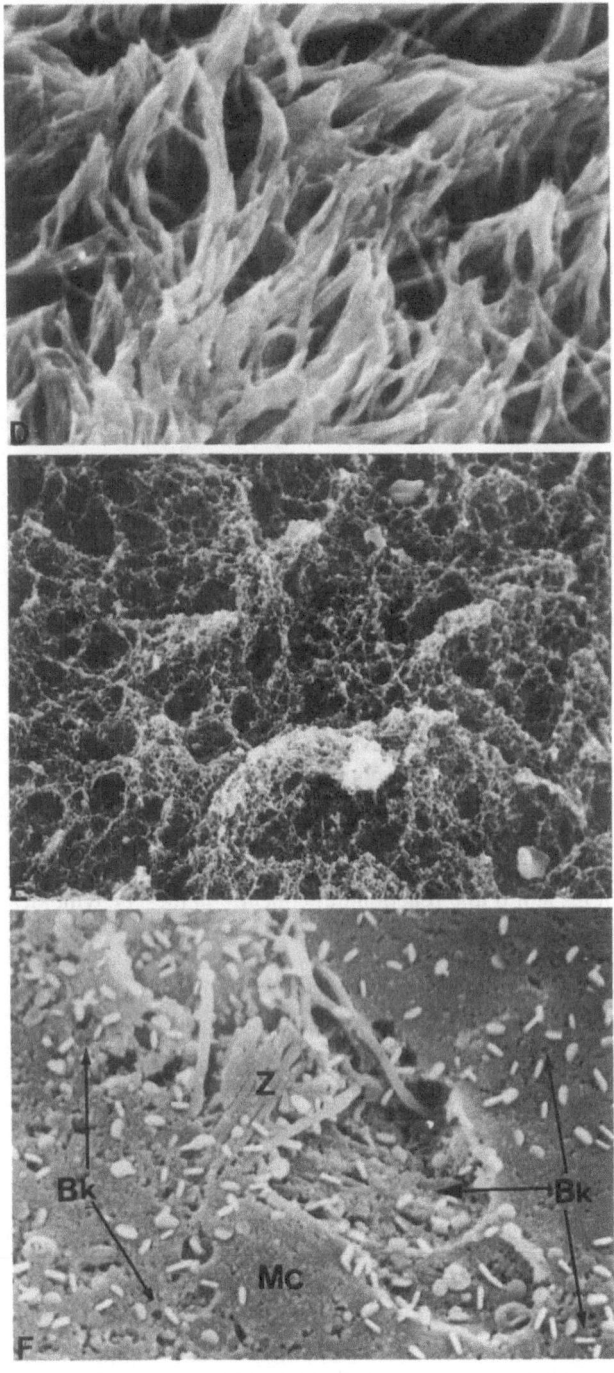

Fig. 2D–F

Summary

Two particularly problematic clinical entities are chosen from the many possible causes of the pathophysiology of subglottic tracheal stenoses in childhood: (a) malformations of the "hard" and "soft" types of stenosis occurring typically as primary lesions; and (b) stenoses caused by trauma (following intubation or faulty tracheostomy) as the most common secondary lesions. It is shown with reference to experimental investigations that subepithelial layers play the leading role in the origin of stenoses, in contrast to hitherto existing ideas based on clinical observations. Traumatic stenoses caused by unphysiological mechanical stressing show striking parallels to those in other age groups, suggesting the conclusion that a reaction of the mesenchymal tissue layers of the airway regions in question is a typical response to mechanical forces.

Résumé

Deux aspects cliniques particulièrement graves des sténoses trachéales subglottiques de l'enfant ont été choisis dans le but d'en éclaircir la physiopathologie: (a) les malformations de type "rigide" et "souple" en tant que lésions primaires caractéristiques et (b) les sténoses dues à des traumatismes (après intubation ou trachéotomie non conforme aux règles de l'art) en tant que lésions secondaires fréquentes. L'étude expérimentale effectuée montre que ce sont les couches sous-épithéliales qui jouent un rôle prépondérant dans l'apparition des sténoses, contrairement à ce que les observations cliniques avaient pu faire croire jusqu'alors. En ce qui concerne les sténoses dues à des traumatismes, donc à des forces mécaniques non physiologiques, on constate qu'elles présentent une parfaite similitude avec les lésions que l'on observe chez les patients d'un âge différent et que par conséquent il s'agit d'une réaction des couches du mésenchyme des voies respiratoires à des forces mécaniques.

Zusammenfassung

Aus der Vielfalt der Entstehungsursachen subglottischer Trachealstenosen im Kindesalter werden zur Erläuterung der Pathophysiologie 2 besonders problematische klinische Erscheinungsbilder herausgegriffen: (a) Mißbildungen in Form der „harten" und „weichen" Stenosen als typische primäre Schäden und (b) traumatisch bedingte Stenosen (postintubatorisch, nach fehlerhafter Tracheotomie) als häufigste Sekundärläsionen. Anhand experimenteller Untersuchungen wird aufgezeigt, daß bei ihrer Entstehung entgegen den bisherigen, vorwiegend auf klinischen Beobachtungen beruhenden Vorstellungen den subepithelialen Gewebsschichten die führende Rolle zufällt. Für die traumatisch bedingten, also auf einer unphysiologischen mechanischen Belastung beruhenden Stenosen ergeben sich dabei auffällige Parallelen zu Krankheitsbildern dieser Region auch anderer Lebensalter, was die Schlußfolgerung nahelegt, daß die Reaktion der mesenchymalen Gewebsschichten eine typische Antwort der fraglichen Luftwegsabschnitte auf mechanische Einwirkungen darstellt.

References

Heineken H (1952) Beitrag zur angeborenen Kehlkopfatresie. Frankfurt Z Pathol 63:30

Kallius E (1897) Beiträge zur Entwicklungsgeschichte des Kehlkopfes. Anat Hefte 9:303

Meyer R (1971) Behandlung der Trachealstenose. Arch Klin Exp Ohr Nas Kehlk Heilkd 199:292

Minnigerode B (1962) Zur Ausbreitung des Plattenepithels im menschlichen Kehlkopf im Hinblick auf die Entstehung der „hellen Flecke" am hinteren Taschenbande. Arch Ohr Nas Kehlk Heilkd 179:290

Minnigerode B (1965) Chorditis vocalis interior hypertrophica (seu hyperplastica). Neue Gesichtspunkte zur pathologisch-anatomischen Einordnung des Krankheitsbildes. Pract Oto-Rhino-Laryngol 27:290

Minnigerode B (1969) Die subglottische Stenose. HNO 17:132

Minnigerode B (1971) Pathophysiologie der Stenosen von Kehlkopf und Trachea. Arch Klin Exp Ohr Nas Kehlk Heilkd 199:65

Minnigerode B, Küpper R (1977) Die chirurgische Behandlung von Larynx- und Trachealstenosen nach translaryngealer intratrachealer Dauerintubation im Kindesalter. Z Kinderchir 22:111

Minnigerode B, Richtering I (1969) Die angeborene partielle subglottische Stenose des Neugeborenen. Z Kinderchir 7:180

Minnigerode B, Richter HG, Bartholomé W (1980) Die Flächenausdehnung traumatischer Schleimhautveränderungen und ihre Bedeutung für die rekonstruktive Chirurgie bei Kehlkopf- und Trachealstenosen nach Langzeitintubation. HNO 28:45

Mounier-Kuhn P, Gaillard I (1962) Le syndrome trachéale. A propos d'une statistique hospitalière. Ann Oto Laryngol 79:159

Padovan I, Orescovic M (1971) Die Behandlung der Stenosen des Larynx. Arch Klin Exp Ohr Nas u Kehlk Heilkd 199:254

Singer L (1933) Die entzündlichen Erkrankungen des Mittelohres und der pneumatischen Hohlräume des Mittelohres: I. Z Hals Nas Ohrenheilkd 32:110

Smith II, Bain AD (1965) Congenital atresia of the larynx. Ann Otol 74:338

Virchow R (1887) Über Pachydermia laryngis. Berl Klin Wochenschr 585

Walender A (1955) The mechanism of origin of congenital malformations of the larynx. Acta Otolaryngol (Stockh) 45:426

Subglottic Stenosis in Newborns After Mechanical Ventilation

M. Marcovich[1], F. Pollauf[1], and K. Burian[2]

Introduction

Once artificial ventilation had become one of the main features of neonatal intensive care, a great many problems occurred in connection with mechanical respiratory support.

A less frequent but even more severe complication was laryngeal trauma following endotracheal intubation (Abbott 1968; Choffat et al. 1975; Downs et al. 1966; Fearon et al. 1966; Goumaz 1973; Hatch 1968; Hawkins 1978; Hengerer et al. 1975; Jones et al. 1981; Lindholme 1970; Mattila et al. 1969; McGovern et al. 1971; Papsidero and Pashley 1980).

Treatment of these acquired − mostly subglottic − stenoses is difficult and may involve hospital treatment lasting several months or even years.

Although the problem is already familiar − it was described as early as 1916 (Turner 1916) − no complete satisfactory method of management has been found so far.

Of course, prevention would be the best method, but the frequency actually seems to have increased during recent years (Hatch 1968; Holinger et al. 1976; Ratner and Whitfield 1983).

As previous studies (Fearon and Cotton 1974; Ratner and Whitfield 1983) emphasize the hazards of a conservative "wait and see" attitude, we have tried to adopt a more aggressive approach to the problem.

Since Holinger (1982) has said, "It seems that any premature infant, full-term infant, or child requiring tracheotomy who is stable and healthy enough to breathe spontaneously and undergo general anaesthesia would be a candidate for the laser procedure", and since Healy et al. (1978) has called the surgical carbon dioxide laser "the single greatest advance in transoral surgery of the airway in the past 15 years, an ideal tool for the infant and juvenile larynx", we chose laser surgery to cope with the problem.

Patients and Methods

From 1979 to 1983 inclusive a total of 854 newborns requiring artificial ventilation were admitted to the Neonatal Department of the Children's Hospital of the City of Vienna, Glanzing.

[1]Neonatal Intensive Care Unit, Children's Hospital of the City of Vienna-Glanzing and [2]Second Department of Otorhinolaryngology, University of Vienna, A-1030 Vienna, Austria.

Progress in Pediatric Surgery, Vol. 21
Ed. by P. Wurnig
© Springer-Verlag Berlin Heidelberg 1987

These patients included five with severe subglottic stenosis in whom extubation was impossible at the end of respirator support, which meant an incidence of 0.6%. One 3-month-old patient was transferred from another neonatal intensive care unit when there was already a clinical suspicion of laryngeal trauma.

The six infants were two girls and four boys. The mean birth weight was 1940 g (1600–2730 g), and the mean gestational age was 34 weeks (32–37 weeks). Ventilator support was required either for hyaline membrane disease (HMD) or for aspiration of amniotic fluid.

Noncuffed, disposable endotracheal tubes (Rüschelit) of the smallest possible size were used; nasotracheal intubation was used, and the patients were ventilated with time-cycled, pressure- or volume-limited respirators.

The mean duration of ventilator support was 42 days (13–87 days) and the mean duration of endotracheal intubation, 156 days (13–291 days) (Table 1).

If repeated attempts at extubation in patients whose spontaneous breathing was already adequate (CPAP +2 cm of water) failed or signs of respiratory distress occurred immediately or within hours whenever the endotracheal tube was removed the clinical diagnosis was confirmed by microlaryngotracheoscopy (Fig. 1).

Before surgery patients received drug therapy including steroids, anti-inflammatory agents and antibiotics. Several attempts at extubation under the influence of heavy sedation and locally applied steroids (sprays) followed. If conservative management failed the patients underwent laser surgery accomplished with a CO_2 laser.

General anaesthesia was performed with jet ventilation to provide an unrestricted view of the area being operated on (Brummitt et al. 1981; Miyasaka et al. 1980; Rita et al. 1983; Zadrobilek et al. 1981).

We tried to avoid tracheostomy or at least to postpone it as long as possible, and only had recourse to it if there was frequent self-extubation or mucus obstruction of the tube, with the attendant repeated risk of hypoxia. In tracheostomized patients a Silastic tube was inserted through the stenosis after laser vaporization

Table 1. Clinical data of six patients with acquired subglottic stenosis

Patient no., sex	Birth weight (g)	Gestational age (weeks)	Diagnosis	Ventilation (days)	Intubation (days)
12, girl	1850	32	HMD	53	70
2, boy (2nd twin)	1600	32	HMD	16	81
3, boy	2070	36	HMD	13	13[a]
4, boy (1st twin)	1680	34	HMD	87	219
5, girl	2730	37	Aspiration	24	260
6, boy	1710	33	HMD	60	291

[a] Underwent emergency tracheostomy.

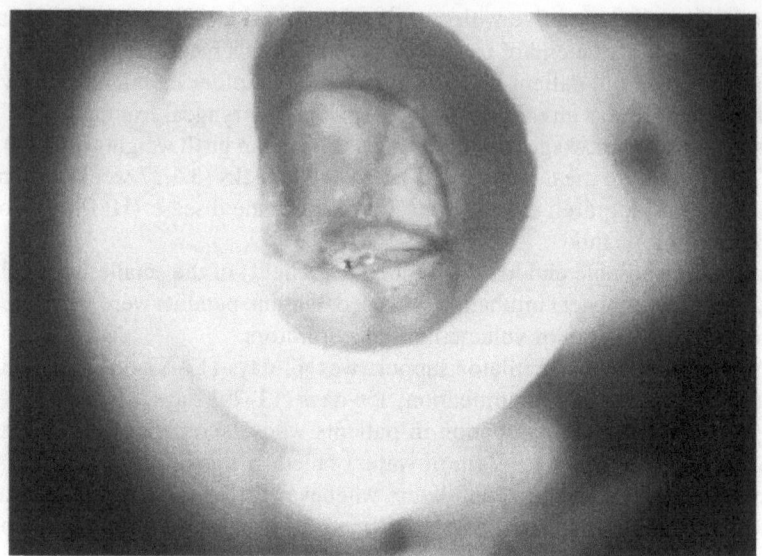

Fig. 1. Severe subglottic stenosis

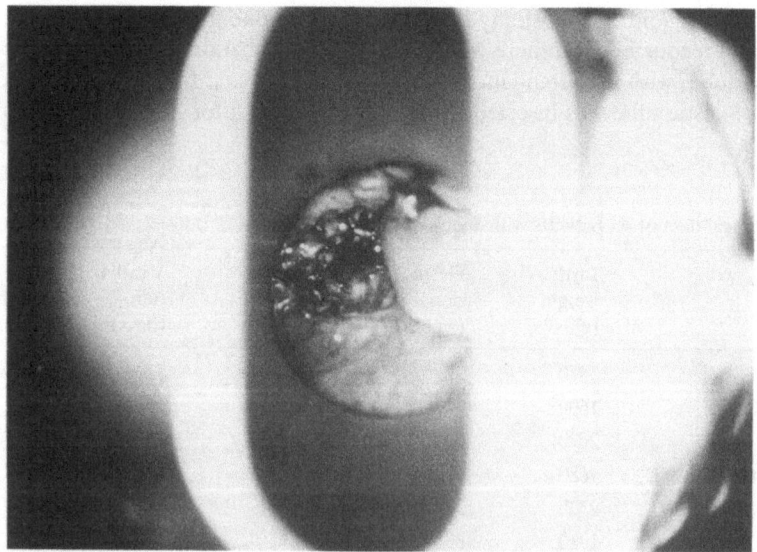

Fig. 2. Treatment of stenosis with laser surgery and Silastic stent

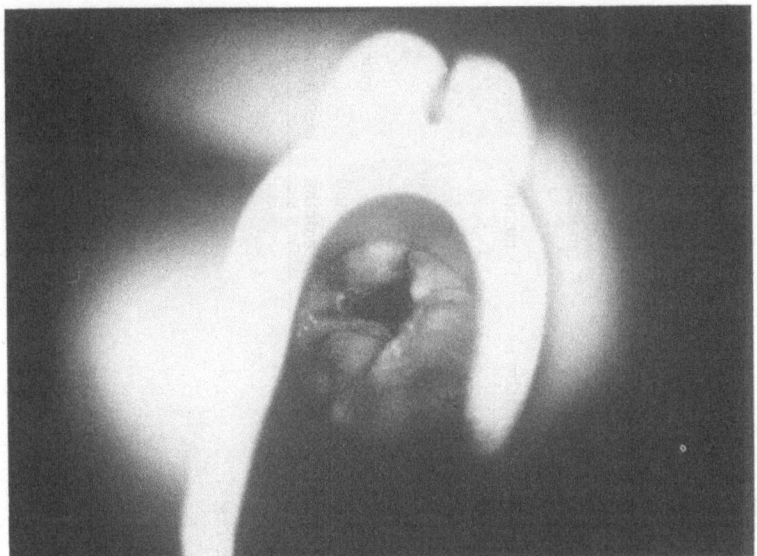

Fig. 3. Adequate airway lumen as a result of correction by laser surgery

of tissue; this acted as a stent and prevented restenosis (Fig. 2). Treatment was continued until a sufficient airway lumen was obtained (Fig. 3).

In addition, a special programme of voice and speech training was developed for tracheostomized children by our speech therapy department (Fleischhacker and Marcovich 1983).

Results

Cases 1 (Girl) and 2 (Boy)

Subglottic stenosis was clinically suspected at the ages of 2 months (case 1) and 2 weeks (case 2), and was confirmed by endoscopy only in case 2.

Both patients were given steroids and anti-inflammatory agents for about 2 weeks. After several attempts at extubation − 6 in case 1 and 15 in case 2 − extubation was finally possible after 2½ months (case 1) and 3 months (case 2). Neither tracheostomy nor surgical intervention was necessary (Table 2).

Case 3 (Boy)

After 13 days of mechanical ventilation extubation was possible without problems. The patient was discharged home in good condition at the age of 6 weeks. One week later readmission was necessary because of sudden airway distress. The patient's mother had already noticed "breathing problems" over the past 2 or 3 days, especially while feeding the baby. As there was almost complete subglottic atresia of the larynx and endotracheal intubation was impossible, emergency

Table 2. Treatment of six patients with acquired subglottic stenosis

	Case no., sex						
	1, girl	2, boy	3, boy	4, boy[a] A	4, boy[a] B	5, girl	6, boy
Age at onset of clinical symptoms	9 weeks	2 weeks	7 weeks	12 weeks	18 months	3 weeks	2 months
Age at endoscopic diagnosis	–	2 months	7 weeks	5 months	18 months	1 month	3 months
No. of extubations efforts	6	15	1	38	6	43	25
Age at first laser surgery	–	–	2½ months	6 months	20 months	1 month	8 months
No. of laser operations	–	–	12	1	3	7	2
Age at tracheostomy	–	–	7 weeks (emergency)	–	20 months	8 months	–
Age at final extubation	2½ months	3 months	–	7 months	–	–	9½ months
Age at decannulation	–	–	2½ years	–	2½ years	Still under therapy	–
Time of stenosis treatment	2 weeks	2½ months	2¼ years	4 months	1 year	Not yet completed	7 months
Time in hospital	3 months	4 months	14 months	12 months	8 months	9 months	8 months

[a] A, first stenosis; B, recurrent stenosis.

tracheostomy had to be performed. Laser surgery was started at the age of 2½ months and a total of 12 operations were performed. Successful decannulation was possible when the patient was 2½ years old (Table 2).

Case 4 (Boy)

Symptoms of subglottic stenosis occurred after prolonged ventilation (87 days) for severe HMD and bronchopulmonary dysplasia. Endoscopy was performed at the age of 5 months. A 7-week period of steroid therapy had no effect and was fol-lowed by laser intervention. Extubation was possible 3 weeks after surgery and the patient was discharged home.

Recurrent airway distress at the age of 18 months necessitated endoscopy. During general anaesthesia with jet ventilation pneumothorax occurred and the patient had to be intubated for resuscitation and intensive care. Once more the endotracheal tube could not be removed at the end of respirator therapy.

Because of repeated self-extubation and tube obstruction the patient had to be tracheostomized at the age of 20 months. Laser surgery was started again, and within 4 months three operations were performed. In addition to tissue excision a Silastic bougie was placed in the stenotic area to prevent restenosis. At the age of 2½ years the patient could finally have the cannula removed (Table 2).

Case 5 (Girl)

This premature girl was our most difficult patient and therapy has not yet been completed. At the age of 1 month, when several extubation efforts had failed, endoscopy of the larynx showed a haemangioma in the subglottic area. Immediate laser excision was performed, but attempts at extubation were not successful. In-creasing nursing problems necessitated tracheostomy at the age of 8 months. At that time several laser procedures had shown no effect. The patient's mother ob-jected to further treatment and the cannulated patient was discharged home. When therapy was started again at the parents' request when the patient was 2½ years old, endoscopy showed a completely atretic subglottic area with a long stenosis. The therapy is still in progress (Table 2).[1]

Case 6 (Boy)

After 2 months of mechanical ventilation patient 6 was admitted from another hospital for treatment of a stenosis. Endoscopic diagnosis at the age of 3 months confirmed inflammation and oedema of the subglottic mucosa. Conservative management with steroids failed. Laser surgery at the age of 8 and 9 months was followed by successful extubation (Table 2).

As surgical experience increased we learned to extend the intervals between operations, so traumatized mucosa had a chance of epithelization between laser events.

Depending on the patient's home situation we tried to discharge the children as soon as possible and to treat them as outpatients. This was only possible if

---

[1] Meanwhile successfully operated.

tracheostomy had been performed. The parents had to be trained for special care while the patients were still in hospital; suction equipment had to be provided for home treatment.

By early use of perforated cannulas and intensive speech therapy we obtained almost normal voice and speech development in five of the patients, thus giving them the chance of normal social integration (Fleischhacker and Marcovich 1983).

All our patients survived and showed excellent physical and mental condition.

Discussion

Many possible factors have been made implicated in the development of subglottic stenosis following endotracheal intubation.

The tube itself, its size, its material (Editorial 1975; Guess and Stetson 1968; Hillman et al. 1975; Mattila et al. 1969; Stetson 1975), the sterilization method used for the tube (Mattila et al. 1969; Stetson 1975), and also a blunt intubation technique, prolonged use of endotracheal tubes associated with up and down movements during ventilation and nursing care, self-extubation and reintubation have all been blamed for tissue irritation and subsequent mucosal trauma.

Analysis of our six cases of subglottic stenosis revealed no significant difference in clinical data or treatment characterizing the patients who developed extubation problems.

Birth weights were not extremely low – as Ratner and Whitfield (1983) reported – nor were any of the patients full-term neonates, whom Hawkins (1978) claimed to be more sensitive to intubation trauma than premature babies.

None of them had suffered especially traumatizing intubation in the delivery room; only well-trained doctors had intubated the newborns, and they had used small disposable noncuffed tubes so any air leak age would be audible. Neither the duration of respiratory support nor the number of times reintubations was accomplished was above average compared with the data of other patients, who often had to withstand much more neonatal stress and did not show any subsequent airway problems.

So, even if we admit the contribution of all factors mentioned above, this does not explain why some intubated infants develop subglottic stenosis while others treated in the same way do not. In addition, use of the terms "prolonged" and "traumatizing intubation" is still at issue. According to some authors (Göcke 1983; Holinger et al. 1976; Turner 1916) laryngeal damage is present even after some hours of intubation, whereas Johnson (1973) reports no subglottic stenosis if intubation does not exceed 6 days.

The incidence of acquired larynx stenosis following endotracheal intubation was extremely high when prolonged intubation started to be used on a wider scale. Frequencies of up to 24% were reported in the 1960s (Fearson et al. 1966), while later studies presented figures between 0.4% and 2.5% (Parkin et al. 1976; Ratner and Whitfield 1983); we found an incidence of 0.6% among our respirated newborns.

Once the problem appears, the possible ways of dealing with it are few: (a) Doing nothing and waiting for the patient to outgrow the problem; (b) conservative management with steroids and dilatation; (c) open surgery; or (d) laser surgery.

The first approach prevailed in earlier years, when any surgical intervention was thought to interfere with the normal growth of the larynx (Jackson and Jackson 1937; Lederer 1943). As patients did not outgrow an acquired subglottic stenosis, but had high tracheostomy, mortality and morbidity rates (Fearon and Cotton 1974; Ratner and Whitfield 1983), the proof that there was no connection between laryngeal surgery and laryngeal development (Calcaterra et al. 1974; Cotton and Evans 1981; Fearon and Cotton 1972, 1974) led to a more active approach. Systemic and local steroid therapy in combination with bougienage did not have satisfactory results (Waggoner et al. 1973). Many surgical techniques with varying degrees of success have been reported (Aboulkar 1968; Cotton 1978; Cotton and Seid 1980; Evans 1975; Evans and Todd 1974; Fearon and Cotton 1972, 1974; Fearon et al. 1978; Grahne 1971; Louhimo et al. 1971; Majeski et al. 1980; Ogura and Spector 1976; Rethi 1956). Cotton and Seid's (1980) method of splitting the cricoid while the newborn is still intubated seems the most promising one, but the question arises as to whether surgery is not performed to early and thus unnecessarily if patients weigh only between 1 and 2 kg at the time of operation. Cotton himself admits that it is possible these infants could have been extubated without surgical intervention.

We decided on the laser method because we wished to avoid tracheostomy as far as possible, and also all complications connected with open surgery, such as bleeding, postoperative oedema, wound infection, and scarring (Mayer et al. 1980; Steiner et al. 1980).

In 1976 Holinger still favoured early tracheostomy after 5–7 days of intubation. Tracheostomy rates of 86% (Ratner and Whitfield 1983) or 97% (Holinger et al. 1976) were reported. Today the hazards connected with tracheostomy – high mortality rates, development of stenosis as a result of the tracheostomy itself – are well recognized, and most workers try to avoid the procedure if possible (Cotton and Seid 1980; Healy et al. 1978; Holinger 1982; Koufman et al. 1981).

Three of our patients had to be tracheotomized. In case 1 this was performed as an emergency procedure when near-complete laryngeal atresia had already occurred at home and reintubation was impossible. In case 2 the primary stenosis had been treated successfully without tracheostomy. Restenosis after 18 months was connected with nursing problems (mucus plugging of the tube, self-extubation) and necessitated tracheostomy 2 months later. In case 3 the patient's mother urged us to discharge the patient for home care and this was only possible with a cannula.

Three patients did well without tracheostomy.

No major problems occurred with laser surgery. We found no anaesthetic complications such as have been reported by other workers (Devries 1980; Hirshman and Smith 1980; Vivori 1980; Vourch and Tannieres 1980), except for one case of pneumothorax, which did not occur in connection with laser surgery but with endoscopy.

Our results are difficult to compare with other reports of laser surgery, because most of the cases analysed deal with older patients or with the problem of congenital subglottic stenoses; but they all present quite promising success rates (Healy et al. 1978; Holinger 1982; Koufman et al. 1981; Krajina 1982; Morgon 1982).

Conclusion

Any kind of oedema or granulation in the subglottic region means restriction of the airway lumen, since outward expansion is prohibited by the cartilaginous ring of the cricoid. The fact that even 1 mm of subglottic swelling reduces the newborn airway to 32% of its normal area (Holinger et al. 1976) demonstrates the dimension of our problem.

In 1974 Fearon and Cotton claimed three criteria for successful management of stenosis: (a) a mortality rate of less than 25%; (b) a success rate of more than 75% with good airway, normal voice and normal laryngeal development; and (c) a treatment period of considerably less than 3 years.

These aims have almost been met in our patients. None of the patients died, and five of the six patients were treated successfully; they have no airway problems, their voices are quite normal, and no signs of laryngeal growth alterations have been noted so far. In all patients but one treatment was completed in less than 3 years.

The approach to subglottic stenosis in newborns should start with conservative steps; it was successful in one third of our patients and spared them any further aggressive procedures.

Only if conservative management fails do we feel that surgical correction is indicated, and we recommend laser surgery.

Regarding earlier reports of high mortality and morbidity in preterm infants with severe acquired subglottic stenosis (Turner 1916), we found it important to present our results and to suggest a possible way of managing this challenging problem.

Summary

Mechanical ventilation in the neonatal period is sometimes followed by difficulty in removal of the endotracheal tube although the patient does not need further respiratory support. This problem results from subglottic stenosis consequent on prolonged use of endotracheal tubes. We found this complication in 5 patients among 854 newborns who required artificial respiration. A further patient was admitted from another hospital because of extubation problems. Our clinical diagnosis was confirmed by endoscopy. Drug therapy with steroids and anti-inflammatory agents was tried in all six patients and was successful in two. In four patients conservative management failed and laser surgery was performed; three of these infants required tracheostomy. In two decannulation has already been performed at the age of 2½ years. In conclusion: five of six patients were treated successfully, and one 3-year-old patient is still being treated.

In the light of reports from other authors, this approach can be recommended for the management of acquired subglottic stenosis.

Résumé

Lorsque la respiration assistée n'est plus nécessaire chez les nouveaux-nés primitivement intubés il est parfois difficile d'enlever le tube. Cela peut être dû à une sténose subglottique par à une mauvaise tolérance à long terme de l'intubation. Cette complication a été rencontrée dans cinq cas parmi 854 cas de respiration assistée de nouveaux-nés. L'un des patients nous venait d'un autre hôpital, précisément à cause de ce problème. Le diagnostic clinique fut confirmé par endoscopie. Tous les patients furent soumis à une thérapeutique par médication, stéroides et substances antiinflammatoires et dans deux cas, elle réussit. Dans les quatre autres cas, il a fallu pratiquer une intervention chirurgicale. Trois de ces enfants subirent une trachéotomie. Deux d'entre eux ont pu être décanulés à l'âge de 2 ans et demi. En résumé, nous pouvons dire que le traitement a été couronné de succès dans cinq cas. Le sicième enfant est toujours en traitement. Il semble que les techniques employées puissent être, en règle générale, recommandées pour le traitement des sténoses trachéales subglottiques.

Zusammenfassung

Nach künstlicher Beatmung in der Neugeborenenperiode kommt es manchmal zu Schwierigkeiten den Endotrachealtubus zu entfernen, obwohl der Patient keiner Beatmung mehr bedarf. Dieses Problem kann von subglottischen Stenosen herrühren, die mit verlängerter Anwendung der Endotrachealtuben einhergehen. Wir fanden diese Komplikation bei 5 von 854 Neugeborenen, die künstlich beatmet werden mußten. Ein Patient wurde uns wegen Extubationsproblemen von auswärts überwiesen. Die klinische Diagnose wurde durch Endoskopie bestätigt. Die medikamentöse Therapie mit Steroiden und Antiphlogistika, die bei allen 6 Patienten versucht wurde, führte bei 2 Patienten zum Erfolg. Bei den übrigen 4 Patienten versagte die konservative Therapie, und es mußte operiert werden. Drei dieser Kinder wurden tracheotomiert, wobei 2 bereits im Alter von 2½ wieder dekanüliert werden konnten. Zusammenfassend kann gesagt werden, daß 5 der 6 Kinder erfolgreich behandelt wurden. Ein Patient steht noch in Behandlung. Auch unter Bezugnahme auf die Angaben anderer Autoren kann das beschriebene Vorgehen zur Behandlung der subglottischen Trachealstenose empfohlen werden.

References

Abbott TR (1968) Complications of prolonged nasotracheal intubation in children. Br J Anaesth 40:347–353

Aboulker P (1968) Traitement des sténoses trachéales. Probl Actuels Otorhinolaryngol 275

Brummitt WM, Fearon B, Brama I (1981) Anesthesia for laryngeal laser surgery in the infant and child. Ann Otol Rhinol Laryngol 90:475–477

Calcaterra TC, McClure R, Ward PH (1974) The effect of laryngofissure on the developing canine larynx. Ann Otol Rhinol Laryngol 83:810–813

Choffat JM, Goumaz CF, Guex JC (1975) Laryngotracheal damage after prolonged intubation in the newborn infant. In: Stetson JB, Swyer PR (eds) Neonatal intensive care. Green, St. Louis, pp 253–270

Cotton R (1978) Management of subglottic stenosis in infancy and childhood. Ann Otol Rhinol Laryngol 87:649–657

Cotton RT, Evans JNG (1981) Laryngotracheal reconstruction in children: five-year follow-up. Ann Otol Rhinol Laryngol 90:515–520

Cotton R, Seid AB (1980) Management of the extubation problem in the premature child: anterior cricoid split as an alternative to tracheotomy. Ann Otol Rhinol Laryngol 89:508–511

Devries P (1980) CO_2 laser: a fire hazard when used in upper airways. Medical Post, November 18, p 2

Downs JJ, Striker T, Stool S (1966) Complications of nasotracheal intubation in children. (Letter to the Editors.) N Engl J Med 274:226

Editorial (1975) Plasticisers and the pediatrician. Lancet 1:1172

Evans JNG (1975) Laryngeal disorders in children. In: Wilkinson AW (ed) Recent advances in pediatric surgery. Churchill Livingstone, New York, pp 174–182

Evans JNG, Todd GB (1974) Laryngotracheoplasty. J Laryngol Otol 88:589–597

Fearon B, Cotton R (1972) Surgical correction of subglottic stenosis of the larynx: preliminary report of an experimental surgical technique. Ann Otol Rhinol Laryngol 81:508–513

Fearon B, Cotton R (1974) Surgical correction of subglottic stenosis of the larynx in infants and children. Ann Otol Rhinol Laryngol 83:428–431

Fearon B, MacDonald RE, Smith C, et al (1966) Airway problems in children following prolonged endotracheal intubation. Ann Otol Rhinol Laryngol 75:975–986

Fearon B, Crysdale WS, Bird R (1978) Subglottic stenosis of the larynx in the infant and child: methods of management. Ann Otol Rhinol Laryngol 87:645–648

Fleischhacker S, Marcovich M (1983) Sprecherziehung bei langzeittracheotomierten Kleinkindern. Sprache-Stimme-Gehör 7/2:63–67

Göcke H (1983) Intubationsschäden in den großen Luftwegen Neugeborener. In: Rügheimer E (ed) Intubation, Tracheotomie und bronchopulmonale Infektion. Springer, Berlin Heidelberg New York Tokyo, pp 45–51

Goumaz CF (1973) Laryngotracheal sequelae of prolonged intubation in newborn infants. ORL J Otorhinolaryngol Rel Spec 35:1–14

Grahne B (1971) Operative treatment of severe chronic traumatic laryngeal stenosis in infants up to three years old. Acta Otolaryngol (Stockh) 72:134–137

Guess WL, Stetson JB (1968) Tissue reaction to organotin-stabilizied polyvinyl chloride (PVC) catheters. JAMA 204:118

Hatch DJ (1968) Prolonged nasotracheal intubation in infants and children. Lancet 1:1272–1275

Hawkins DB (1978) Hyaline membrane disease of the neonate, prolonged intubation in the management: effects on the larynx. Laryngoscope 88:201–224

Healy GB, McGill T, Strong MS (1978) Surgical advances in the treatment of lesions of the pediatric airway: the role of the carbon dioxide laser. Pediatrics 61:380–383

Hengerer AS, Strome M, Jaffe BF (1975) Injuries to the neonatal larynx from long-term endotracheal tube intubation and suggested tube modification for prevention. Ann Otol Rhinol Laryngol 84:764–770

Hillman LS, Goodwin SL, Sherman WR (1975) Identification and measurement of plasticiser in neonatal tissues after umbilical catheters and blood products. N Engl J Med 292:381

Hirshman CA, Smith J (1980) Indirect ignition of the endotracheal tube during carbon dioxide laser surgery. Arch Otolaryngol 106/10:639–641

Holinger LD (1982) Treatment of severe subglottic stenosis without tracheotomy. Ann Otol Rhinol Laryngol 91:407–412

Holinger PH, Kutnick SL, Schild JA, Holinger LD (1976) Subglottic stenosis in infants and children. Ann Otol Rhinol Laryngol 85:591–600

Jackson C, Jackson CL (1937) The larynx and its diseases. Saunders, Philadelphia, p 188

Johnson S (1973) What is prolonged intubation? Acta Otolaryngol (Stockh) 75:377–378

Jones R, Bodnar A, Roan Y, et al (1981) Subglottic stenosis in newborn intensive care unit graduates. Am J Dis Child 135:367–368

Koufman JA, Thompson JN, Kohut RI (1981) Endoscopic management of subglottic stenosis with the cosub 2 surgical laser. Otolaryngol Head Neck Surg 89/2:215–220

Krajina Z (1982) Esperienza sull'uso del laser in laringologia. Acta Otol Rhinol Laryngol 2:99

Lederer FL (1943) Diseases of the ear, nose and throat. Davis, Philadelphia, p 657

Lindholme CE (1970) Prolonged endotracheal intubation. Acta Anaesthesiol Scand [Suppl] 33:1–131

Louhimo I, Grahne B, Pasila M, et al (1971) Laryngotracheal stenosis in children. J Pediatr Surg 6:730–737

Majeski JA, Schreiber JT, Cotton R, MacMillan BG (1980) Surgical correction of tracheal stenosis in the pediatric burn patient. J Trauma 20:81–86

Mattila MA, Suutarinen T, Sulamas M (1969) Prolonged endotracheal intubation or tracheostomy in infants and children. J Pediatr Surg 4:674–682

Mayer T, Matlak ME, Dixon J, et al (1980) Experimental subglottic stenosis: histopathologic and bronchoscopic comparison of electrosurgical, cryosurgical, and laser resection. J Pediatr Surg 15/6:944–952

McGovern FH, FitzHugh GS, Edgemon LJ (1971) The hazards of endotracheal intubation. Ann Otol Rhinol Laryngol 80:556–564

Miyasaka K, Sloan IA, Froese AB (1980) An evaluation of the jet injector (Sanders) for bronchoscopy in paediatric patients. Can Anaesth Soc J 27:117–124

Morgon A (1982) Uso del laser in laringologia pediatrica. Acta Otol Rhinol Laryngol 2:121

Ogura JH, Spector CJ (1976) Reconstructive surgery of the larynx and laryngeal part of the pharynx. Scientific foundation of otolaryngology. Year Book Medical Publishers, Chicago, pp 894–919

Papsidero MJ, Pashley NR (1980) Acquired stenosis of the upper airway in neonates: An increasing problem. Ann Otol Rhinol Laryngol 89:512–514

Parkin JL, Stevens MH, Jung AL (1976) Acquired and congenital subglottic stenosis in the infant. Ann Otol Rhinol Laryngol 85:573–581

Ratner I, Whitfield J (1983) Acquired subglottic stenosis in the very-low-birth-weight infant. Am J Dis Child 137:40–43

Rethi A (1956) An operation for cicatricial stenosis of the larynx. J Laryngol Otol 70:283–293

Rita L, Seleny F, Holinger FD (1983) Anesthetic management and gas scavenging for laser surgery of infant subglottic stenosis. Anesthesiology 58/2:191–193

Steiner W, Jaumann MP, Pesch HJ (1980) Endoskopische Laserchirurgie im Larynx. Ther Umsch 37/12:1103–1109

Stetson JB (1975) The safety testing of tracheal devices. In: Stetson JB, Swyer PR (eds) Neonatal intensive care. Green, St. Louis, pp 271–287

Turner AL (1916) Stenosis of the larynx in children following intubation and tracheotomy. J Laryngol Otol 31:313

Vivori E (1980) Anaesthesia for laryngoscopy. Br J Anaesth 52:638

Vourch G, Tannieres ML (1980) L'anesthesie pour la microchirurgie laryngee sous laser. A propos de 665 cas. Anesth Analg Reanim 37/5–6:339–340

Waggoner LG, Belenky WM, Clark CE (1973) Treatment of acquired subglottic stenosis. Ann Otol Rhinol Laryngol 82:822–826

Zadrobilek E, Draxler V, Riegler R, Höfler H (1981) Injektbeatmung bei direkter Laryngoskopie und endolaryngealen mikrochirurgischen Eingriffen in Allgemeinanaesthesie. Anaesthesist 30:191–195

Treatment of Congenital Cricoid Stenosis

R. N. P. Berkovits[1], E. J. van der Schans[1], and J. C. Molenaar[2]

Introduction

Congenital stenosis of the cricoid is a rare malformation which has generally proved fatal up to now. Excessive cartilage causes narrowing of the lumen of the larynx, which leaves only a hairlike canal posteriorly. In severe congenital cricoid stenosis the child usually develops respiratory distress shortly after birth. In the case of a slight occlusion of the larynx, this may only become apparent on exertion or during an upper airway infection. In most cases an emergency tracheostomy has to be performed because of acute infection of the upper airway. Diagnosis is confirmed with the aid of direct laryngoscopy and laryngography.

Materials and Methods

Between 1971 and 1986 a total of seven patients presented with congenital cricoid stenosis at the Sophia Children's Hospital in Rotterdam. There were five boys and two girls. Tracheostomy was required in all of them. The age at tracheostomy varied from a few hours after birth to 2 years of age. The patients were all examined with the aid of direct laryngoscopy and laryngography. The lateral view at laryngography proved the most important diagnostic aid. Once the diagnosis had been confirmed a submucous correction was carried out, followed by prolonged nasotracheal intubation. The first three patients in this series have already been reported elsewhere (Berkovits et al. 1978). We have developed a surgical procedure which has proved very effective. Except for the first case, all our patients underwent this procedure.

Surgical procedure

A laryngofissure is created. The solid cricoid cartilage is split like an apple in the front midline until the posterior hairlike canal is reached. By blunt dissection the mucous membrane is dissected free from the cranial and caudal aspects of the cartilaginous obstruction. The operation is performed as a microsurgical procedure under 10 times magnification, which allows scrupulous preservation of all mucous

[1]Department of Otorhinolaryngology and [2]Paediatric Surgery, University of Rotterdam, Sophia Children's Hospital, NL-Rotterdam, The Netherlands.

membranes. A curved gouge is used to remove the excess cartilage, except for a small, anterior portion which is preserved for subsequent reconstruction of the cricoid ring. The mobilized mucous membrane is then closed with Dexon 5/0. No cricoid cartilage is left exposed. Finally, a solution of methylprednisolone acetate (40 mg) and hyaluronidase (300 IU) is injected into the subglottic region to prevent excessive scar tissue formation. The cannula previously introduced at tracheostomy is then removed and nasotracheal intubation is initiated. This intubation is generally required for approximately 7 weeks. The tubes are changed every 2 weeks and corticosteroids and hyaluronidase are injected at the same time.

Equipment

The gouge was specially designed (R.N.P.B.) to achieve the correct curvature. Our intubation material consisted of silicone rubber tubes, also especially designed for the purpose (R.N.P.B.) and manufactured to our specifications. The material is very soft, approximately 35 shore. In comparison, ordinary silicone rubber endotracheal tubes are 50–70 shore. The material is nontoxic, as substantiated in tissue culture tests (Berkovits 1971). The tubes are submerged in silicone oil (20 cSt). Impregnation results in a 60% increase in weight as the oil is absorbed by the tube. Friction tests on these impregnated tubes demonstrated extremely good friction properties, comparable with the friction of ice on ice (Berkovits et al. 1978). During intubation the oil will seep out slowly and continuously in small quantities, creating a system of boundary and weeping lubrication. Direct contact of mucous membrane with the intubation material is thus avoided, while mucus cannot adhere to the tube due to the film of silicone oil. Recovery and growth of mucous tissue is promoted owing to the combination of low-friction, nontoxic and extremely pliable material, correct sizing of the tube avoiding pressure not only on the mucous membranes but also on the underlying tissues. Such optimal conditions will even enable the treatment of severe iatrogenic damage to an airway (Bos et al. 1973).

Patients

In our first case we used an endolaryngeal approach to the cricoid stenosis. This patient was a 1-month-old girl who had been progressively dyspnoeic from birth, requiring an emergency tracheostomy on 13 January 1971. The diagnosis of cricoid stenosis was confirmed by laryngography (Fig. 1a).

On 15 March 1971 she was operated upon, and the cartilaginous obstruction was removed via an endolaryngeal approach. Postoperatively she was intubated nasotracheally for 26 weeks, with a change of tubes every week. Corticosteroids and hyaluronidase were injected every 3 weeks.

The remaining six patients all underwent the same surgical procedure as described above. The first one (our second case) was a 2-year old boy. His respira-

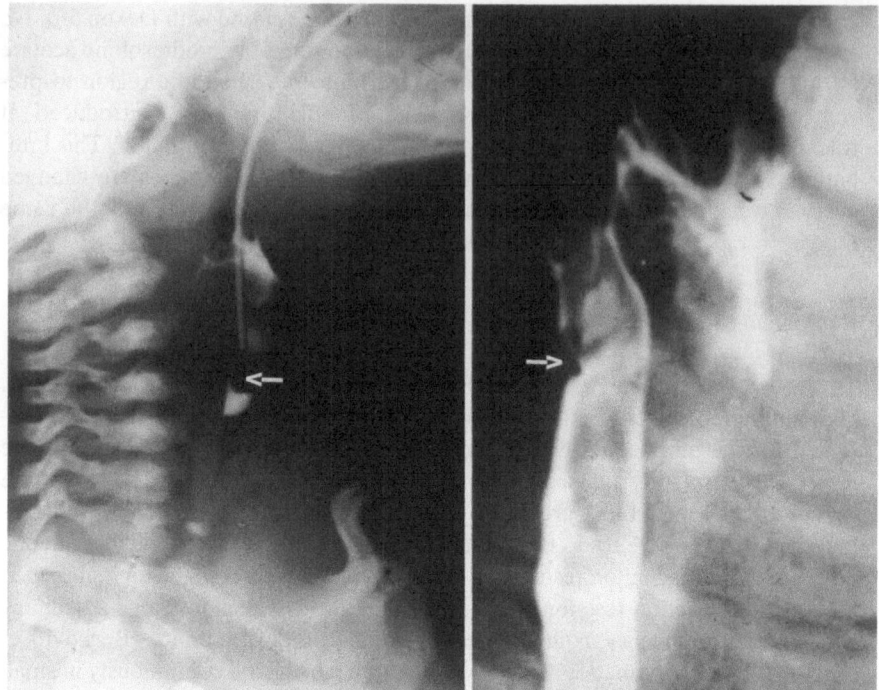

a   b

Fig. 1a, b. Laryngograms of the first patient. **a** Preoperative characteristic narrowing of the subglottic area; note the wedge-shaped, thick cricoid cartilage *(arrow)*. **b** Lateral film of the neck showing normal subglottic space postoperatively, with only a slight irregularity of the ventral wall *(arrow)*

tion had been audible from birth, occasionally developing into stridor. He presented with an acute respiratory infection an 20 May 1976, requiring emergency tracheostomy. Laryngoscopy and laryngography revealed the classic subglottic obstruction caused by excessive cricoid cartilage, in this case leaving a canal with a diameter of 3 mm sagitally (Fig. 2).

Operation followed a month later. This patient was the first to undergo laryngofissure, and the operative procedure was photographed. Figure 3a provides a good view of the obstructive cartilage still in situ, which has been removed in Fig. 3b. The 1.5-mm catheter introduced at tracheostomy is clearly visible in the posterior canal.

The duration of postoperative nasotracheal intubation was 4 weeks, and in this case the tubes were changed once a week.

The special merit of laryngography as a diagnostic technique was demonstrated in our third patient. This boy had also had audible respiration from birth and presented with acute respiratory infection at 5 months of age, requiring emergency tracheostomy in August 1976. Direct laryngoscopy revealed *total*

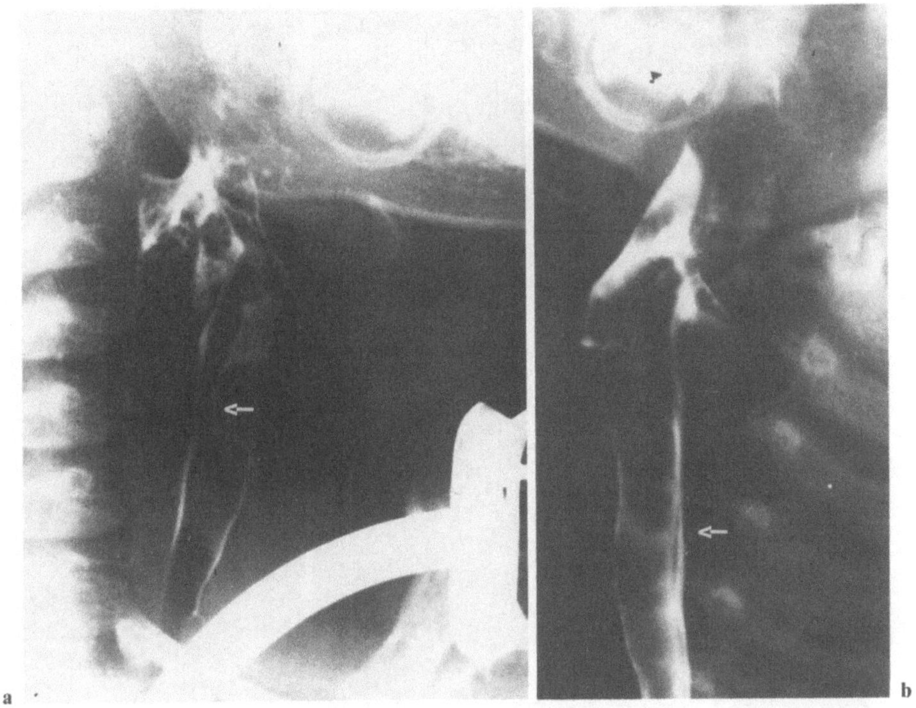

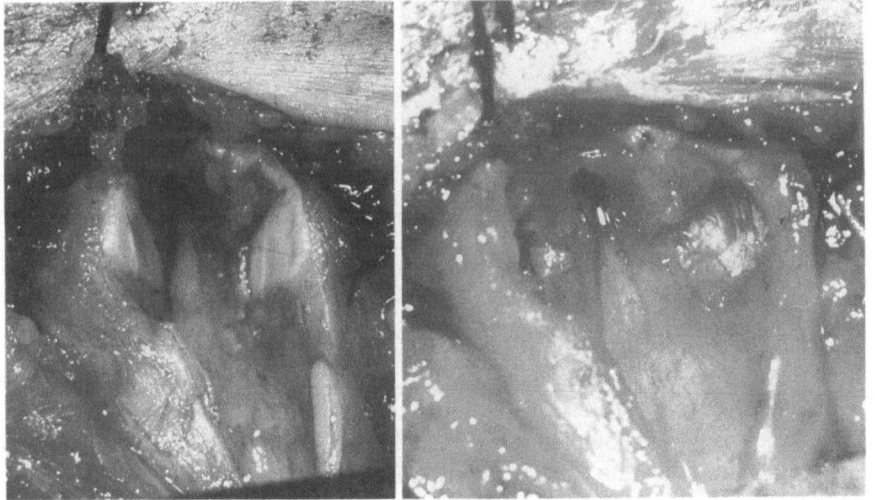

Fig. 2a, b. Laryngograms of the second patient. **a** Preoperative obstruction *(arrow);* **b** laryngo-tracheography showing a normal airway postoperatively at the site of the previous obstruction

Fig. 3a, b. Preoperative photographs taken of patient 2, showing laryngofissure. **a** The obstructive cartilage is clearly visible; **b** same site after removal of excessive cartilage

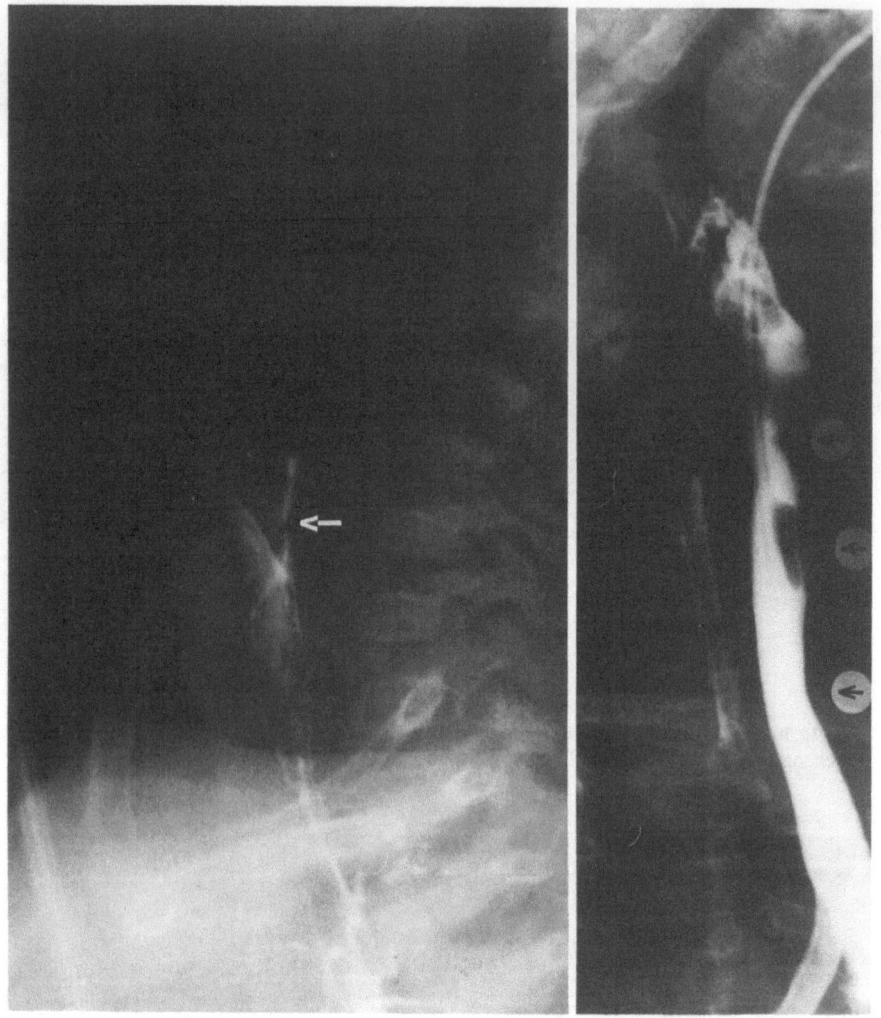

Fig. 4a, b. In case 3 preoperative laryngography was performed through the tracheostomy (**a**); the *arrows* indicate the severe obstruction of the airway. A lateral laryngogram (**b**) taken 3 months after surgery reveals only slight narrowing on the site of the previous obstruction

obstruction at the level of the vocal cords. Laryngography performed through the tracheostomy revealed the characteristic picture of congenital cricoid stenosis, with a hairlike canal posteriorly, although in this case the occlusion was extreme. The vocal cords were completely obstructed as a result of a forceful but unsuccessful attempt at intubation carried out elsewhere (Fig. 4).

Of the remaining four patients, three boys and one girl, two presented in 1978, one in 1981 and one in 1983. All four required emergency tracheostomy shortly after birth, at ages ranging from 5 h to 1 month. By then our surgical regimen had

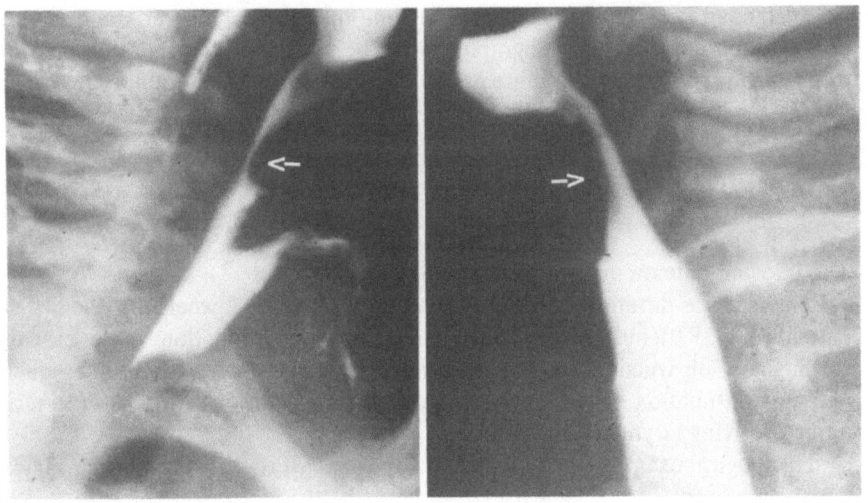

Fig. 5. Lateral laryngogram of patient 4, showing classic obstruction before correction
Fig. 6. Lateral laryngotracheogram of patient 5, showing characteristic localization of obstructive cartilage

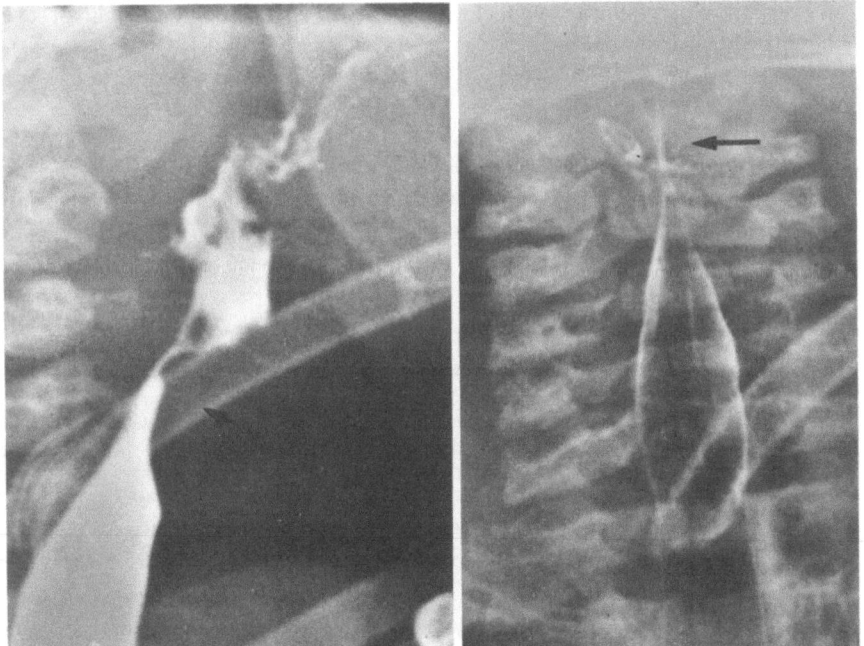

Fig. 7a, b. Laryngotracheography of patient 6. **a** Lateral view, clearly showing site of obstruction and extent of occlusion. **b** Front view; obstruction is not seen very clearly

been standardized, and they all underwent the surgical procedure described above. In two of them laryngography had to be performed through the tracheostomy. Figures 5–7 illustrate these cases. The superiority of lateral laryngography as a diagnostic aid is clearly demonstrated in Fig. 7.

Results

The relevant data on our patients are shown in Table 1.

The average duration of nasotracheal intubation was 7 weeks for the last six patients only. Patient 1 required an extended period of intubation. In this case the cartilaginous obstruction was removed endolaryngeally. In view of the subsequent extensive intubation, this technique proved clearly inferior to the surgical technique involving laryngofissure.

Histological examination of the excessive cartilage revealed normal cartilaginous tissue.

The follow-up period varies from almost 6 months to 15 years at the time of writing. In all seven patients respiration has remained unobstructed following extubation. Postoperative laryngography showed a normal airway, although in some cases a slight irregularity of the ventral wall or a slight narrowing on the site of the previous obstruction persisted (see Figs. 1b, 2b, 4b). Postoperatively, none of these patients has shown any signs of respiratory distress, either while at rest or on exertion. Consequently, we feel we have achieved a complete cure in all seven patients.

Discussion

Apart from our series of seven patients, no more than fourteen cases of congenital cricoid stenosis have been described in the literature; only five of these were treated successfully (Morimitsu et al. 1981). In a retrospective, post-mortem study

Table 1. Details of seven patients treated for congenital cricoid stenosis in 1971–1986

Patient no.	Sex	Age at tracheostomy	Age at surgery	Duration of intubation	Follow-up	Outcome
1	F	1 month	3 months	26 weeks	15 years	Cured
2	M	2 years	2 years	4 weeks	11 years	Cured
3	M	6 months	7 months	8 weeks	10 years	Cured
4	M	1 month	2 months	8 weeks	8 years	Cured
5	F	14 days	1½ years	10 weeks	7½ years	Cured
6	M	5 hours	8 months	6 weeks	5½ years	Cured
7	M	1 month	11 months	2 months	2½ years	Cured

reported in 1962, Potter diagnosed only three cases out of a total of well over 6000 neonates. Subsequently, Smith and Bain reported nine cases in 1965, when they also reviewed all cases reported up to then. According to their information, this anomaly was first described by Rossi in 1826. In view of our comparatively large number of cases and the numbers reported by Smith and Bain, we surmise that this congenital malformation occurs more frequently than is generally assumed.

Our experience with these seven patients demonstrates that a laryngofissure is essential in the surgical correction of congenital cricoid stenosis. Microsurgical removal of the obstructive cartilage should be combined with prolonged naso-tracheal intubation. In this connection it is imperative to use only nontoxic, low-friction intubation material, such as the silicone rubber tubes described above.

The results obtained with our surgical procedure using the specially designed intubation material demonstrate the effectiveness. We feel this method consti-tutes a major advance not only in the treatment of congenital cricoid stenosis, but also in the treatment of iatrogenically damaged airways.

Acknowledgments. The intubation material was kindly supplied to our specification by Lubrelas-tic Medical Appliances, Hazerswoude, Holland. We are indebted to Dr. M. Meradji, paediatric radiologist, for his invaluable radiological expertise. Alice Goslinga Ribbink, translater/stylistic editor, is thanked for preparing the manuscript.

Summary

Congenital cricoid stenosis is a rare malformation generally diagnosed at autopsy. Out of a total of fourteen cases reported by others, only five were treated success-fully. Over a 10-year period, seven patients presented with congenital cricoid stenosis at the Sophia Children's Hospital in Rotterdam. On the basis of these numbers we surmise that this anomaly is less rare than is commonly thought. All seven patients were treated successfully. A new method of treatment is described, consisting of a combination of microsurgical laryngofissure and prolonged intuba-tion with a new, low-friction, atoxic, soft, silicone rubber nasotracheal tube. The specially designed intubation material is also recommended for the treatment of iatrogenically damaged airways. The results indicate that this method constitutes a major advance not only in the treatment of cricoid stenosis but also in the treat-ment of damaged airways.

Résumé

La sténose congénitale du cricoïde est une malformation rare dont le diagnostic est posé, en règle générale, lors de la nécropsie. Parmi les 14 cas mentionnés par d'autres auteurs, 5 seulement ont été traités avec succès. Au cours d'une période de 10 ans, 7 patients présentant une sténose congénitale du cricoïde ont été traités à l'hôpital des enfants Sophia à Rotterdam. C'est pourquoi nous pensons que cette malformation est plus fréquente qu'on ne le croit généralement. Les 7 patients ont tous été traités avec succès. On décrit une nouvelle méthode qui con-siste à combiner une laryngofissure par microchirurgie et une intubation pro-longée avec un nouveau tube nasotrachéal en silicone qui glisse très bien, est non toxique et souple. Ce tube de fabrication spéciale est recommandé également pour le traitement des lésions des voies respiratoires iatrogéniques. Les résultats indiquent que cette méthode offre des avantages considérables non seulement pour le traitment de la sténose du cricoïde mais aussi dans le cas d'autres lésions des voies respiratoires.

Zusammenfassung

Die kongenitale Krikoidstenose ist eine seltene Fehlbildung, die gewöhnlich bei der Autopsie diagnostiziert wird. Von 14 Fällen, die von anderen Autoren berich-tet wurden, konnten nur 5 erfolgreich behandelt werden. In einem 10-Jahreszeit-raum kamen 7 Patienten mit kongenitaler Krikoidstenose am Sophia-Kinderkran-kenhaus in Rotterdam zur Behandlung. Aufgrund dieser Zahl nehmen wir an, daß diese Fehlbildung häufiger ist als gewöhnlich angenommen wird. Alle 7 Pa-tienten wurden erfolgreich behandelt. Eine neue Behandlungsmethode wird be-schrieben, die aus einer Kombination von mikrochirurgischer Laryngofissur und verlängerter Intubation mit einem neuen, leichtgleitenden, atoxischen, weichen Silikonnasotrachealtubus besteht. Dieser speziell hergestellte Tubus wird auch für die Behandlung iatrogener Luftwegsläsionen empfohlen. Die Resultate sprechen dafür, daß diese Methode große Vorteile nicht nur in der Behandlung der Krikoid-stenose, sondern auch in der Behandlung anderer Luftwegsläsionen bringt.

References

Berkovits RNP (1971) Therapeutische laryngotracheale intubatie. Doctoral thesis, Rotterdam
Berkovits RNP, Bos CE, Pauw KH, De Gee AW (1978) Congenital cricoid stenosis. Patho-genesis, diagnosis and method of treatment. J Laryngol Otol 92:1083–1100
Bos CE, Berkovits RNP, Struben WH (1973) Wider application of prolonged nasotracheal intu-bation. J Laryngol Otol 87:263–280
Morimitsu T, Matsumoto I, Okada S, Takahashi M, Kosugi T (1981) Congenital cricoid stenosis. Laryngoscope 91:1356–1364
Potter E (1962) Pathology of the fetus and infant. Year Book Medical Publishers, Chicago, p 310
Smith II, Bain AD (1965) Congenital atresia of the larynx. Ann Otol Rhinol Laryngol 74: 338–349

Surgical Correction of Laryngotracheal Stenoses in Children

E. Hof[1]

Introduction

Laryngotracheal stenoses are increasing in frequency owing to the advances in anaesthesiology and neonatology, giving even newborns with severe respiratory problems a chance of survival. Thus, congenital malformations of the laryngo-tracheal region are dealt with, but acquired stenoses are then observed (Banfai 1976; Tucker 1975, 1978). Sooner or later a tracheostomy becomes necessary in either congenital or acquired stenosis. A small child with a tracheal cannula, how-ever, is exposed to disturbances in general development, and the cannula is also an enormous burden, both physically and psychiologically, for the whole family. Therefore, the earliest possible removal of cannulas in such children has been a major aim for some years in Zurich.

Patients and Method

A total of 63 children with laryngotracheal stenoses or anomalies are the subjects of this study. Most of them were operated on in Zurich (starting in 1973) and some by invitation at the Paediatric Surgical Hospital of the Dr. von Haunersches Kinderspital of the University of Munich (starting in 1982). Five children pre-sented with extreme congenital laryngeal anomalies (Table 1). After birth they had to undergo emergency tracheostomy since intubation was not possible. Three children had congenital bilateral paralysis of the vocal cord which had unfortu-

Table 1. Aetiology of laryngotracheal stenoses in children

Aetiology	No. of cases
Laryngeal anomalies	5
Subglottic stenoses	54
Subglottic stenoses and paralysis of the vocal cord	4

[1] Otorhinolaryngology Clinic, University Hospital of Zurich and University Children's Hospital, CH-8091 Zurich, Switzerland.

Progress in Pediatric Surgery, Vol. 21
Ed. by P. Wurnig
© Springer-Verlag Berlin Heidelberg 1987

nately not been diagnosed (Hof 1984). These children remained intubated for a long time and developed subglottic stenosis in addition. Acquired stenoses resulted from long-term intubation, traumatic intubation or high-pressure ventilation in 54 children. The youngest child to be operated on was 14 months old and the oldest 12 years; the oldest child had previously undergone irradiation of a mediastinal lymphoma. The average age of the children at operation was 2.9 years.

Operative Technique

The operative technique described by Rhéti in 1959 for widening of the upper airways was modified. The principle of our technique, as in Rhéti's method, is dilatation of the cricoid, which is entirely transected ventrally and dorsally (Figs. 1–7). The operative field is clearly exposed via a T-shaped skin incision above the

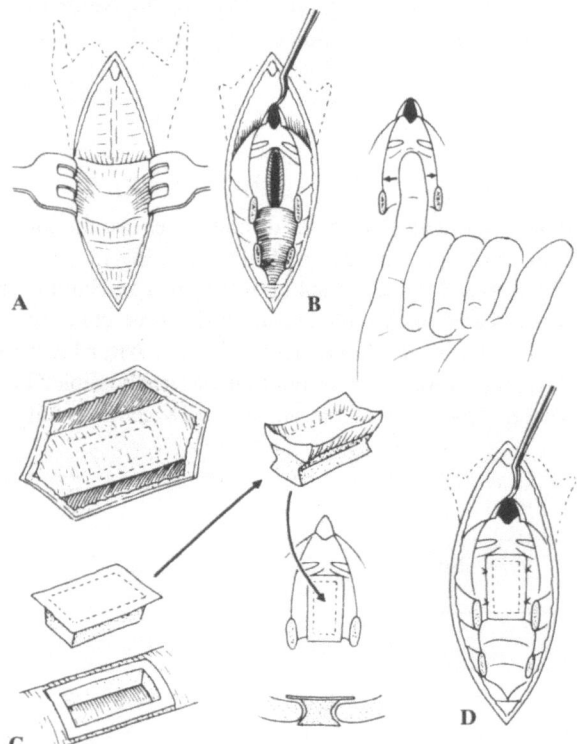

Fig. 1A–D. Schematics showing aspects of the operation. **A** Exposure of the trachea and the subglottic region; **B** transection of the anterior tracheal wall and the posterior cricoid, followed by digital palpation to make sure that the entire stenosis has been removed; **C** costal cartilage notched laterally to fit exactly in the separated cricoid and trachea; **D** costal cartilage inserted in the separated posterior cricoid

Figs. 2–6. Course of the Operation

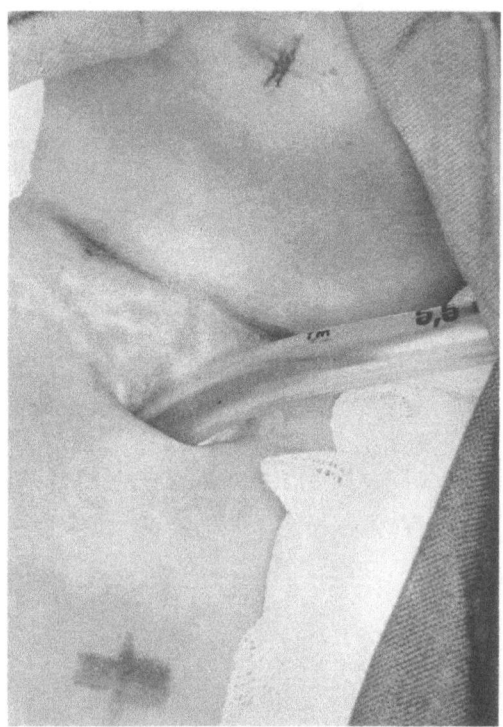

Fig. 2. T-shaped skin incision above tracheostomy

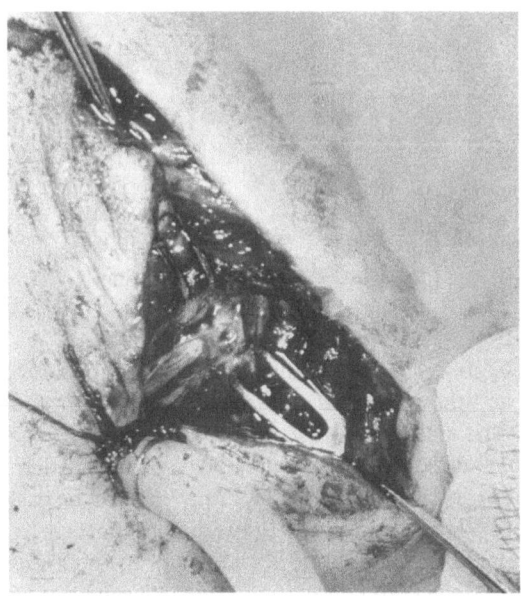

Fig. 3. Costal cartilage put in the separated posterior cricoid

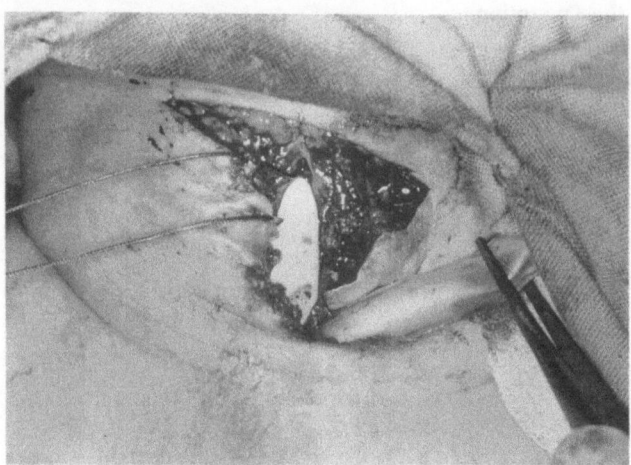

Fig. 4. Insertion of the splintin tube

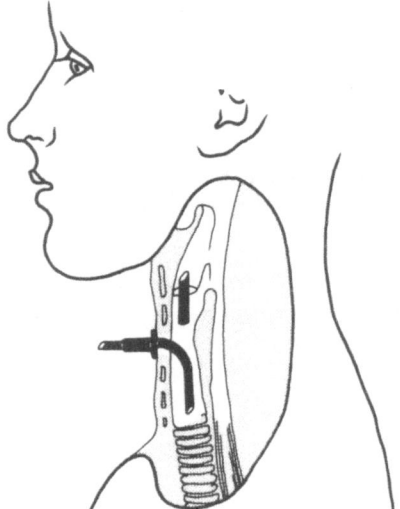

Fig. 5. Schematic of upper splinting tube and lower tracheal cannula for ventilation

thyroid cartilage and trachea. The lower rim of the thyroid cartilage is transected up to the anterior commissure and the incision is continued through the cricoid and the first two tracheal rings. The anterior halves are separated, thus exposing the posterior cricoid wall, which is subsequently transected and also separated. A piece of costal cartilage resected in advance is notched laterally so it can be easily wedged in the transected and separated posterior wall of the cricoid. Further fixation is achieved by a splinting tube, which is inserted at the end of the operation, and extends from 3 mm above the vocal cord nearly to the tracheal cannula. This

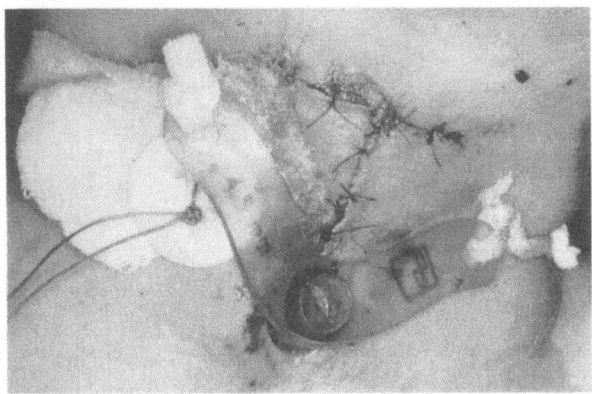

Fig. 6. Fixation of the splinting tube by means of transcutaneous suture and support button

tube is fixed by a suture leading to the exterior. The T-shaped tubes used in adults are not suitable for small children. The splinting tube remains in place for 6–8 weeks and is then removed endolaryngeally. Experience shows that subsequently granulations develop in the area of the operation, which must be repeatedly resected endolaryngeally until decannulation is possible, usually 6 months after surgery.

Results and Discussion

Forty-eight children were decannulated an average of 6 months after surgery (Table 2). A slightly deep, hoarse voice resulted in all children, which was, however, easily understandable. There have been no respiratory problems even in the children who were decannulated over 10 years ago. Four children had to undergo re-operation for recurrent stenosis. In one child we had to perform first a laryngoplasty and then a vocal cord operation for laryngotracheal stenosis and abduction of the vocal cord. Only after both these procedures could the child be decannulated. Among the 10 children in whom we have to regard the results as failures, there were three deaths, which were not, however, directly related to surgery. One boy died of obstruction of the tracheal cannula after removal of the splinting tube when he had been referred to his home hospital. The boy with previously irradiated lymphoma and subsequent tracheal stenosis could be decannulated within 1 year after surgery. However, he developed recurrence of the stenosis requiring a further tracheostomy and died 4 years postoperatively from pneumonia developing from massive bronchiectases. Three children were primarily transferred for operation for subglottic stenosis. Preoperative tracheoscopy, however, revealed the formerly unrecognized diagnosis of paralysis of the vocal cord, which had necessitated long-term intubation with subsequent stenosis. In these three children the stenosis had to be repaired before the vocal cord operation could be

Table 2. Results of 63 laryngotracheoplasties

	Decan-nulated	Failure	Death
Laryngotracheoplasty	48	5	2
Repeat operation	4		
Laryngotracheoplasty + vocal cord abduction	1	2	1

performed. One of these children died from pneumonia 6 months after successful laryngotracheoplasty, before the vocal cord operation could be done. The other two children were operated on for vocal cord paralysis. However, decannulation is not yet possible because of recurrent stenosis. Four recently treated children developed major granulations or recurrent stenosis, and further operations are planned in these patients.

Note Added in Proof. Since this paper was prepared a further 23 children have been operated on. This makes a total of 86 children up to August 1986, in 73 of whom laryngeal plasty has been successful.

Summary

A modified surgical technique according to Rhéti is described: the cricoid and the uppermost tracheal rings are longitudinally dissected ventrally and dorsally. The enlargement of the lumen is stabilized by interposition of a notched piece of costal cartilage into the dissected posterior wall of the cricoid. A total of 63 children with laryngotracheal stenosis have been operated on by this method in Zurich since 1973 and in Munich since 1982. Laryngotracheal plasty is successful in over 80% of small children in whom the procedure is necessary. The voice becomes a little hoarse, but respiration is adequate, as demonstrated by our juvenile patients, some of whom have been decannulated for over 10 years. The earlier opinion that laryngoplasty performed in small children might impair laryngeal growth and result in severe stenoses has been disproved by the results presented. Our experience shows that prognosis is worse in children with tracheal stenosis and associated anomalies, such as paralysis of the vocal cord.

Résumé

On décrit une méthode d'intervention chirurgicale selon Rhéti modifiée. Le cartilage cricoïde et les anneaux supérieurs de la trachée sont fendus ventralement et dorsalement sur toute la longueur. On stabilise la dilatation de la lumière en plaçant une greffe chondrocostale dans la fente dorsale du cartilage cricoïde. Depuis 1973 à Zurich et 1982 à Munich, 63 enfants en tout, présentant une sténose laryngotrachéale ont été opérés selon cette méthode. Dans 80% des cas, la reconstitution laryngotrachéale est couronnée de succès chez les petits enfants. La voix reste un peu rauque mais la respiration est satisfaisante ainsi que le prouvent les enfants décanulés, depuis plus de 10 ans pour certains. L'opinion avancée autrefois et selon laquelle une laryngoplastie pratiquée dans la petite enfance empêcherait la croissance du larynx et causerait une sténose grave ulterieure est nettement réfutée par nos résultats. Les enfants qui présentent une sténose trachéale associée à d'autres malformations telles que parésie des cordes vocales par exemple, ont d'après notre expérience, un pronostic beaucoup plus reserve.

Zusammenfassung

Es wird eine modifizierte Operationsmethode nach Rhéti beschrieben. Dabei werden das Krikoid und die obersten Trachealspangen vorne und hinten längs gespalten. Durch Interposition eines gekerbten Rippenknorpelstücks in die gespaltene Krikoidhinterwand wird die gewonnene Lumenerweiterung stabilisiert. Mittels dieser Methode konnten seit 1973 in Zürich und seit 1982 auch in München insgesamt 63 Kinder mit Laryngotrachealstenosen operiert werden. Eine Laryngotrachealplastik beim Kleinkind führt in über 80% zum Erfolg. Die Stimme wird etwas heiser, die Atmung ist jedoch suffizient, wie auch unsere teils schon über 10 Jahre dekanülierten Kinder bestätigen. Die früher geäußerte Meinung, daß eine im Kleinkindesalter ausgeführte Larynxplastik das weitere Wachstum des Kehlkopfes beeinträchtigt und zu schweren Stenosen führt, können wir anhand der vorliegenden Ergebnisse widerlegen. Kinder mit Trachealstenosen, die zusätzliche Mißbildungen wie z. B. Stimmbandparesen aufweisen, haben anhand unserer Erfahrung eine schlechtere Prognose.

References

Banfai P (1976) Die operative Lösung der laryngo-trachealer Stenosen. HNO 24:371
Cryxdale WS (1976) Extended laryngofissure in subglottic stenosis. J Otolaryngol 5/6:479
Hof E (1978) Ergebnisse der operativen Versorgung laryngo-trachealer Stenosen. HNO 26:60
Hof E (1984) Beidseitige kongenitale Abduktionsparesen. ORL 8:69
Rhéti A (1959) Chirurgie der Verengungen der oberen Luftwege. Thieme, Stuttgart
Tucker JA (1975) Some aspects of fetal laryngeal development. Ann Otol 84:49
Tucker JA (1978) Clinical correlation of anomalies of the supraglottic larynx with the staged sequence of normal human laryngeal development. Ann Otol 87:636

Surgical Treatment
of Congenital Laryngotracheo-oesophageal Cleft

R. N. P. Berkovits[1], N. M. A. Bax[2], and E. J. van der Schans[1]

Introduction

Fissure of the dorsal side of the larynx is a rare anomaly, which was first described in 1792 by Richter.

Cotton and Schreiber reviewed the literature in 1981 and found a total of 60 cases documented in the English-language literature. We report four cases, two of which have been reported previously (Berkovits et al. 1974). The first two patients were operated on via a lateral pharyngotomy, and the other two, via an anterior approach.

MacIntosh et al. (1954) studied the occurrence of congenital anomalies in nearly 6000 neonates. Anomalies of the respiratory system were found in 0.2%. Patients with laryngeal fissure were not present in these series. It has therefore been concluded that this anomaly is exceedingly rare.

Petterson (1955) distinguished three degrees of severity:

Type I: Laryngo-oesophageal fissure where only the cricoid is split;
Type II: Laryngotracheo-oesophageal fissure extending up to the four proximal tracheal rings;
Type III: Complete laryngotracheo-oesophageal fissure extending to the carina.

Pathogenesis

The cricoid cartilage probably develops from the sixth branchial arch, and during the sixth week of pregnancy it appears as two lateral areas of cartilage that fuse ventrally and dorsally (Delahunty and Cherry 1969). The tracheo-oesophageal septum arises from two longitudinal ridges in the tracheo-oesophageal groove, which then fuse in a caudocranial direction. Blumberg et al. (1965) assumed that laryngotracheo-oesophageal fissure was caused by premature arrest of the cranial movement of this septum.

Diagnosis

Children with congenital laryngeal clefts choke on every attempt at feeding and frequently suffer from aspiration pneumonia. A weak cry is often described.

[1]Department of Otorhinolaryngology, University of Rotterdam, Sophia Children's Hospital, NL-Rotterdam, The Netherlands.
[2]Department of Paediatric Surgery, Wilhelmina Children's Hospital, NL-Utrecht, The Netherlands.

Progress in Pediatric Surgery, Vol. 21
Ed. by P. Wurnig
© Springer-Verlag Berlin Heidelberg 1987

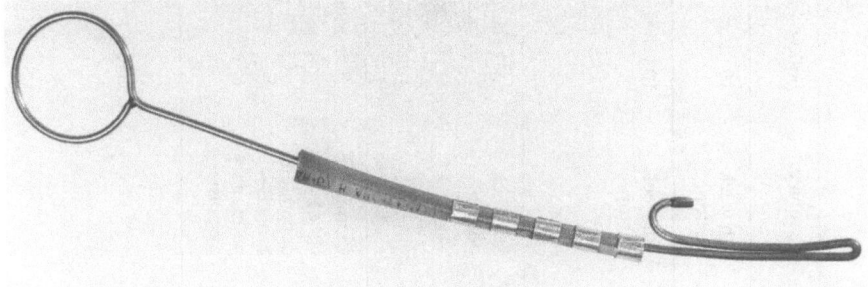

Fig. 1. Probe used to measure laryngotracheo-oesophageal clefts

Cine-oesophagography sometimes reveals (massive) overflow of the contrast agent into the larynx and trachea during the act of swallowing. Therefore a contrast agent suitable for bronchography should be used.

A survey of the literature, and this is backed up by our own experience, shows that the anomaly is often and easily overlooked during endoscopy (Berkovits et al. 1978; Blumberg et al. 1965; Calcaterra et al. 1974; Cotton and Schreiber 1981; Delahunty and Cherry 1969), because skilful introduction of a bronchoscope of the right size fails to separate, and thus to visualize, the cleft. It is therefore important to consider this diagnosis in children with dysphagia and with aspiration pneumonia of puzzling origin. The probe (Fig. 1) described by Berkovits et al. (1965) is useful for diagnosing and measuring the length of the cleft.

Prognosis

Congenital laryngotracheo-oesophageal cleft (CLEC) has a very high mortality. Lim et al. (1979) reported that only patients with type I could survive without surgery. Nevertheless, half the type-I patients died when no repair was done. Surgery is mandatory for type-II and type-III CLEC. Only one patient has been reported to survive type-III CLEC (Ruder and Glaser 1977).

Prognosis is worsened in types II and III by the multiple congenital defects that frequently accompany the clefts.

Case Reports

General information on the patients is given in Table 1.

Patient 1 (Male, 03-02-1968)

A detailed report on this patient has been published elsewhere (Berkovits et al. 1974). Soon after delivery the patient aspirated during feeding and was sub-

Table 1. Patient data

Patient	Sex	Age at diagnosis	Extent of cleft	Concurrent abnormalities	Age at operation	Technique	Extubated	Follow-up
1 (03-02-68)	M	4 mo.	14 mm 3 rings	None	6 m	Left lateral pharyngotomy	4th week postop.	16 years
2 (21-02-72)	M	10 mo.	25 mm 3 rings	Opitz' syndrome Tracheomalacia	13 m	1st: Gastrostomy 2nd: Left lateral pharyngotomy	6th week postop.	10 years
3 (10-06-82)	M	1 mo.	15 mm	Oesophageal atresia Duodenal atresia Severe tracheo-malacia	9 m	(Anterior) laryngofissure	8th week postop.	3½ years
4 (19-01-84)	F	6 wk.	15 mm	Oesophageal atresia and fistula Coloboma Ear deformity Genital deformity	21 m	(Anterior) laryngofissure	Cannula CPAP-dependent broncho-pulmonary dysplasia	8 months

sequently fed by gastric tube. Aspiration pneumonia necessitated an emergency tracheostomy. Only after repeated laryngoscopy at the age of 4 months was a CLEC revealed. The length of the cleft was measured and was 14 mm, as confirmed by cineradiography. Closure of the cleft was accomplished by left lateral pharyngotomy at the age of 18 months. The cleft affected three tracheal rings. A cicatricial subglottic stenosis developed, which was treated with prolonged nasotracheal intubation for 28 days.

The patient was last seen in March 1984. Respiration and feeding presented no problems. The voice was normal. Indirect laryngoscopy revealed paralysis of the left vocal cord in the intermediate position. Expiratory peak flow was in accordance with age and weight.

Patient 2 (Male, 21-02-1972)

This patient was born after a 34-week pregnancy. He had a great many congenital abnormalities, fitting the description of Opitz' syndrome. Oral feeding was instantly complicated by aspiration and aspiration pneumonia. The larynx was considered normal as this point, though the trachea showed signs of malacia. Tracheostomy was performed 5 months after birth.

Repeated laryngoscopy revealed the cleft 10 months after birth. The cricoid cartilage was separated posteriorly between the arytaenoid cartilages, and our probe was used to measure the length of the cleft, which was 25 mm or three tracheal rings. This is a type-II cleft (Petterson).

Tracheoscopy revealed tracheomalacia along the entire length of the trachea, with bulging of the pars membranacea. The bronchoscope could be passed through the upper trachea into the oesophagus.

Before surgical correction of the cleft a gastrostomy was performed. Surgical correction of the cleft was performed at the age of 13 months via a left lateral pharyngotomy. Two weeks postoperatively the tracheostomy cannula was removed. Respiration was mildly obstructed due to tracheomalacia, and after 5 days nasotracheal intubation was performed with a siliconized silicone rubber tube. The child could be extubated after an intubation of 3 weeks.

One year after closure of the cleft oral feeding was started successfully, and the child was discharged 3 months later.

The child was last seen in good condition at the age of 11 years, with a slight tendency to upper airway infections and tracheobronchitis. Laryngotracheo-oesophagoscopy was performed, showing an adequate airway with a closed cleft. The left recurrent nerve was paralysed.

Patient 3 (Male, 10-06-1982)

This patient was delivered by caesarian section after a 34-week pregnancy; birth weight was 2000 g. The congenital pathology was extensive:

1. Combined oesophageal atresia and tracheo-oesophageal fistula. This fistula was corrected on the day of birth.

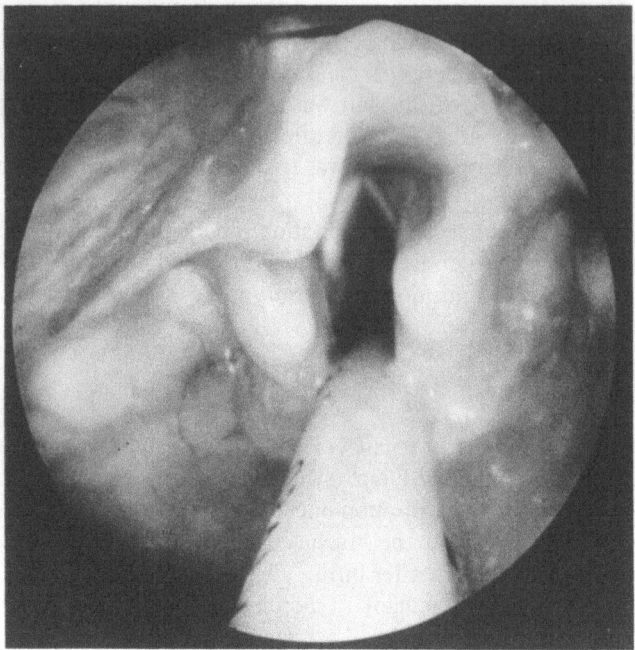

Fig. 2. Endoscopy of cleft. Tube slips posteriorly between arytaenoid cartilages

2. Duodenal atresia; this was corrected 1 week after birth.
3. Tracheomalacia and laryngotracheo-oesophageal cleft of 15 mm (Fig. 2).

Nasotracheal intubation was performed. At the age of 9 months the child was operated on via the anterior approach. The cleft included three tracheal rings. Postoperatively the patient was intubated for 8 weeks. The tube was replaced every 2 weeks. One months after extubation the patient was discharged from hospital.

The patient is doing well to date, 3½ years after treatment. Feeding and respiration present no difficulties. The voice is clear.

Patient 4 (Female 19-01-84)

This child was born prematurely after a 35-week pregnancy. An extensive congenital syndrome was found:

1. Oesophageal atresia with tracheo-oesophageal fistula was corrected on the day of birth
2. CLEC, diagnosed at endoscopy at 6 weeks
3. Coloboma iridis
4. Ear deformity
5. Genital deformity

The patient was fed via a jejunostomy. At the age of 3½ months a laryngofissure was performed with closure of the cleft. Decannulation has not been possible due to serious respiratory problems resulting from bronchopulmonary dysplasia. Endoscopic examination of the larynx has shown that the cleft is closed but the larynx is seriously obstructed by redundant mucosal folds of the posterior wall. The poor general condition of the child has prevented adequate treatment of this obstruction by means of nasotracheal intubation (see description of surgical treatment).

Description of the Surgical Treatment

Anterior Approach

The thyroid cartilage, the cricoid cartilage, and the top four tracheal rings were fissured in the midline. Exposure of the CLEC was excellent (Fig. 3), and surgical manipulation easy. The edges of the cleft were found to be covered by redundant mucosa. The mucosal edges of the cleft were incised and trimmed. The cleft was closed in two layers with gauge 4-0 Vicryl up to the level of the vocal cords (Fig. 4). No stent was placed in the laryngeal lumen.

The skin was closed and a Jackson-type silver tracheostomy cannula left in place.

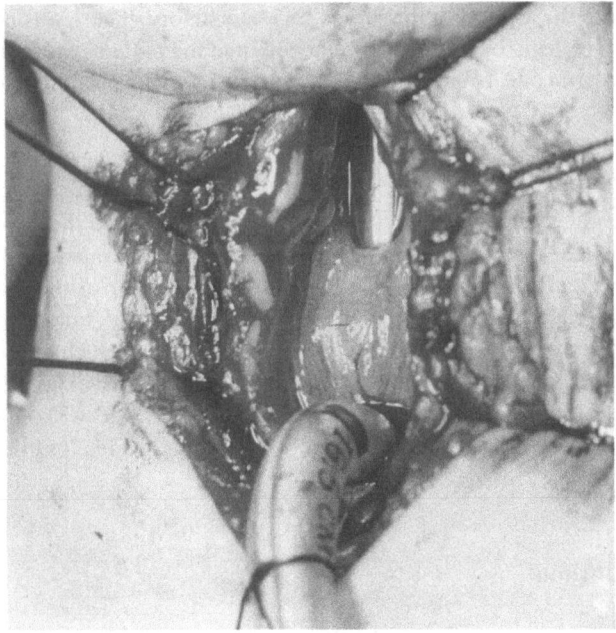

Fig. 3. Exposure of type II cleft via anterior laryngofissure

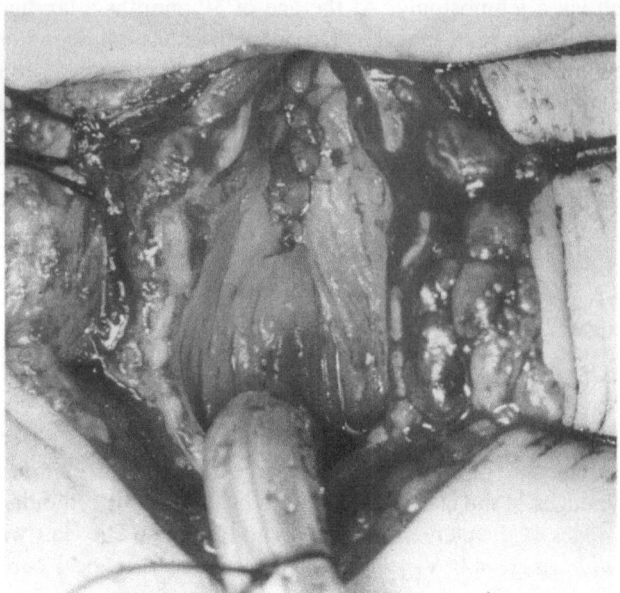

Fig. 4. Closure of cleft completed via laryngofissure

On the 10th postoperative day a laryngoscopy was performed. Wound healing on the posterior and anterior aspects of the larynx was satisfactory. There was no granulation tissue. The tracheostomy tube was removed, and the patient was intubated with a siliconized silicone rubber tube with 3.5 mm i.d. and 6.5 mm o.d. This tube was replaced every 2 weeks and remained in place for 8 weeks.

Left Lateral Pharyngotomy

The child was placed in the supine position with the head turned toward the right shoulder and slightly flexed. A vertical incision was made from the sternal part of the clavicle to the upper part of the larynx along the anterior border of the left sternomastoid muscle. Trachea and oesophagus were identified and tunnelled out, with retraction of the major vessels laterally. The pharynx and as much of the oesophagus as was deemed necessary were opened and the defect thus exposed. The exposed tracheal, laryngeal and oesophageal defects were closed with silk sutures after freshening of the edges. The pharynx and the wound were closed in layers.

Discussion and Conclusions

The anterior approach, first described by Jahrsdoerfer et al. (1967), has certain advantages, the greatest of which is the easy exposure of the defect, which can be precisely closed in layers up to the posterior commissure between the arytaenoid cartilages.

This easy exposure allows precise trimming of the oesophageal mucosa. We believe that the persisting flaccid stenosis of the larynx in patient 4 does not discredit the method. The surgeon who is keen on preserving the tissues is apt to trim the mucosal folds too conservatively, resulting in voluminous mucosal folds obstructing the larynx. The same risk is involved with the lateral approach, and probably even more so. Adequate trimming is essential to prevent bulging of excessive tissue into the airway. It is therefore wise to check the amount of trimming by means of intraoperative direct laryngoscopy, because both too liberal and too conservative trimming can lead to postoperative stenosis.

Important structures, such as the superior and recurrent laryngeal nerves, are not endangered with the anterior approach.

Two possible disadvantages of the anterior approach are impaired stability of the larynx and trachea and adverse effects of a laryngofissure on development of the larynx. The follow-up of our two CLEC patients is short. However, our experience in five patients with a congenital cricoid stenosis successfully operated on by laryngofissure since 1976 gives us confidence in this respect. The effect of laryngofissure on the developing canine larynx was studied by Calcaterra et al. (1974). Caution is needed in interpretation of the results of animal experiments with reference to humans. However, the results of Calcaterra et al.'s study also suggest that the infant larynx may be carefully divided by a midline vertical thyrotomy without impairment of laryngeal development or function.

The only advantage of the lateral approach is that it does not compromise laryngeal stability. On the other hand, this technique is difficult, and exposure is not as good as that obtained by the anterior approach, especially in the upper part of the cleft. According to Cotton and Schreiber (1981), the lateral approach is more suitable for larger clefts. This seems to us a doubtful conclusion, as we believe that ring 4 can be reached via an anterior tracheofissure. For larger clefts (type III) a thoracotomy is inevitable.

A lateral pharyngotomy jeopardizes the laryngeal nerves. Our patients 1 and 2 each had recurrent laryngeal nerve paralysis. Furthermore, the superior laryngeal nerve can be injured with the lateral approach. The resultant deprivation of the sensory side of the cough reflex would make aspiration problems even greater.

Pracy and Stell (1974) advocate posterior pharyngotomy, as was also used by Imbrie and Doyle (1969). Pracy and Stell operated on one patient with this method. Exposure of the CLEC in this way is very difficult, and in our opinion this approach offers no advantages.

After operation cicatricial stenosis of the subglottic region necessitated long-term maintenance of a tracheostomy. Subglottic stenosis of this kind, which occurred in all our patients, was successfully treated in three of our four patients with therapeutic nasotracheal intubation. The fourth patient is still being treated.

In patients 2 and 3 tracheobronchomalacia made prolonged therapeutic nasotracheal intubation necessary. The treatment of tracheomalacia with prolonged intubation (up to 1 year) is effective in our clinical experience, as it was in patients 2 and 3. The association of CLEC and tracheomalacia is not uncommon.

In the nasotracheal intubation technique (Bos et al. 1973) we use tubes made of silicone rubber impregnated with silicone oil (dimethyl polysiloxane) with a viscosity of 20 cSt. The silicone rubber absorbs 60% by weight of the oil. A small quantity of this oil is slowly and constantly seeping out of the tube. A direct contact of the mucous membranes of the airway and the surface of the tube is thus avoided. This situation creates a system that is referred to in engineering as "boundary and weeping lubrication". Friction measurements on these tubes proved them to be of very low friction quality (Berkovits et al. 1978). The tubes are extremely soft (30–40 shores). The impregnated silicone rubber was tested in tissue culture with human fibroblasts and proved to be nontoxic. All these factors, together with a judicious choice of the right size of tube, lessen the likelihood of intubation trauma. Humidification of the tube with a continuous infusion of saline is mandatory (Bos et al. 1973). After 2 weeks the lubricating properties of the tube deteriorate. Therefore, the nasotracheal tube is changed fortnightly.

Our four patients support the view expressed in the literature that the diagnosis is difficult (Blumberg et al. 1965; Cotton and Schreiber 1981; Delahunty and Cherry 1969; Festen et al. 1973; Pracy and Stell 1974). Diagnosis was made at 16 months in patient 1, at 10 months in patient 2, at 1 month in patient 3, and after 21 months in patient 4 (see Table 1). This despite the fact that all patients were examined repeatedly by experienced laryngoscopists.

Acknowledgements. The silicone rubber silicone oil-impregnated tubes were kindly supplied to our specifications by Lubrelastic Medical Appliances, Hazerswoude-Rijndijk, The Netherlands. The illustrations were prepared by the Audio-Visual Department of the Erasmus University, Rotterdam, The Netherlands.

Summary

Laryngotracheo-oesophageal cleft has been considered a rare congenital anomaly, diagnosed when there is respiratory distress on feeding, associated with multiple congenital disorders. A tracheo-oesophageal fistula should be excluded. Diagnosis, even in skillful endoscopic hands, is difficult.

Different approaches to surgical repair have been advocated in literature. Most authors prefer the lateral approach. Only 7 patients have reportedly been treated via the anterior approach. The anterior approach offers the advantage of excellent and also easy exposure of the anomaly. The theoretical disadvantage of postoperative laryngeal instability is not substantiated by experimental work (Calcaterra, Ann Otol 83:810–813, 1974), nor by our own clinical experience in six juvenile patients who underwent laryngofissure for other reasons. A further advantage of the anterior approach is that the laryngeal nerves are not jeopardized as in the lateral approach.

We have treated 4 patients. Two patients have been treated succesfully via a lateral pharyngotomy approach; each of them has a left recurrent nerve palsy. The other two patients were treated via a laryngofissure, one of them successfully;

in the other patient the cleft has been closed with success, but the larynx is still stenosed by excessive mucous membrane folds.

Cicatricial subglottic stenosis, which may occur postoperatively, and the frequently coinciding tracheomalacia, have been successfully treated with prolonged nasotracheal intubation with siliconized silicone rubber tubes. Four patients were treated succesfully. Three other patients have come to our attention. As is often the case, this disorder seems to occur more frequently than was previously thought.

Résumé

La fissure laryngotracheo-œsophagienne est une malformation congénitale rare, accompagnée le plus souvent par un grand nombre d'autres malformations et qui se manifeste par des troubles de la respiration pendant les tétées. Il faut écarter la possibilité d'une fistule tracheo-œsophagienne. Le diagnostic est très difficile même pour ceux d'entre nous qui sont particulièrement adroits en endoscopie.

Diverses techniques opératoires ont été décrites dans la littérature et la plupart des auteurs ont une préférence pour l'abord latéral. Dans 7 cas seulement on a préféré l'abord antéreur qui a l'avantage d'exposer très nettement et facilement l'anomalie. Quant à l'inconvénient théorique d'une instabilité du larynx après l'intervention, il n'a été constaté ni dans notre expérience (Calcaterra, Ann Otol 83:810–813, 1974) ni dans le cas des 6 jeunes gens qui ont subi une laryngofissure pour d'autres raisons. Un autre avantage de l'accès antérieur est que les nerfs du larynx ne risquent pas d'être touchés, comme cela peut être le cas avec l'accès latéral.

Nous avons traité 4 patients. Deux d'entre eux ont subi une pharyngotomie latérale couronnée de succès; les deux ont une paralysie du nerf récurrent. Les deux autres ont subi une laryngofissure, l'un deux avec succès. Dans le cas de l'autre patient, la fente a bien été fermée mais le larynx reste sténosé par un excès de muqueuse.

Nous avons traité avec succès une sténose subglottique cicatricielle qui peut apparaître après l'intervention et qui est souvent accompagnée d'une malacie, par intubation prolongée avec des tubes de silicone. Nous avons traité avec succès 4 patients et nous avons entendu parler de trois autres enfants. Il semblerait donc que cette malformation n'est pas aussi rare qu'on le pensait jusqu'alors.

Zusammenfassung

Die laryngotracheoösophageale Spalte ist eine seltene kongenitale Fehlbildung, meist kombiniert mit multiplen kongenitalen Störungen, die durch Atemnot beim Füttern diagnostiziert wird. Eine tracheoösophageale Fistel sollte ausgeschlossen werden. Die Diagnosesicherung ist selbst in versierten endoskopischen Händen schwierig.

Verschiedene Operationsmethoden sind in der Literatur beschrieben worden, wobei die meisten Autoren den lateralen Zugang bevorzugen. Nur bei 7 Patienten wurde von einem anterioren Zugang berichtet. Der anteriore Zugang bietet den Vorteil einer sehr guten und einfachen Darstellung der Anomalie. Der theoretische Nachteil einer postoperativen Larynxinstabilität konnte im Experiment nicht nachgewiesen werden (Calcaterra, Ann Otol 83:810–813, 1974), ebenso nicht durch unsere eigene Erfahrung bei 6 jugendlichen Patienten, bei denen eine Laryngofissur aus anderen Gründen durchgeführt wurde. Ein weiterer Vorteil ist der, daß beim anterioren Zugang die Larynxnerven nicht gefährdet werden, wie es beim lateralen Zugang der Fall ist.

Wir behandelten 4 Patienten. Zwei Patienten wurden erfolgreich über eine laterale Pharyngotomie operiert; bei beiden blieb eine Rekurrensparese. Die beiden anderen wurden über die Laryngofissur operiert, einer davon erfolgreich; beim anderen Patienten wurde zwar die Spalte erfolgreich verschlossen, jedoch ist der Larynx noch durch massive Schleimhautfalten stenosiert.

Eine narbige subglottische Stenose, die postoperativ auftreten kann, und die häufig damit kombinierte Tracheomalazie wurden erfolgreich mit verlängerter nasotrachealer Intubation mittels silikonierter Silikontuben behandelt. Wir behandelten 4 Patienten erfolgreich und erfuhren von 3 weiteren behandelten Kindern, so daß diese Fehlbildung doch häufiger vorzukommen scheint als früher angenommen.

References

Berkovits RNP, Bos CE, Struben WH, Vervat D, Van Es HW (1974) Congenital laryngotracheo-esophageal cleft. Arch Otolaryngol 100:442–443

Berkovits RNP, Bos CE, Pauw KH, DeGee AWJ (1978) Congenital cricoid stenosis. Pathogenesis, diagnosis and method of treatment. Laryngol Otol 92:1083–1100

Blumberg JB, Stevenson JK, Lemire RJ, Boyden EA (1965) Laryngo-tracheoesophageal cleft, the embryologic implications: Review of the literature. Surgery 57:559–566

Bos CE, Berkovits RNP, Struben WH (1973) Wider application of prolonged nasotracheal intubation. J Laryngol Otol 87:263–279

Calcaterra TC, McClure R, Ward PH (1974) Effect of laryngofissur on the developing canine larynx. Annals Otol Rhinol Laryngol 83:810–813

Cotton RT, Schreiber JT (1981) Management of laryngotracheoesophageal cleft. Ann Otol Rhinol Laryngol 90:401–405

Delahunty JE, Cherry J (1969) Congenital laryngeal cleft. Ann Otol Rhinol Laryngol 78:96–106

Festen C, Van den Broek P, Marres EHMA (1973) De laryngo-orcheo-oesophageale fissur. Ned Tijdschr Geneeskd 117:1006–1010

Imbrie JD, Doyle PJ (1969) Laryngotracheoesophageal cleft. Report of a case and review of the literature. Laryngoscope 79:1252–1274

Jahrsdoerfer RA, Kirschner JA, Thaler SU (1967) Cleft larynx. Arch Otolaryngol 86:108–113

Lim TA, Spanier SS, Kohut RI (1979) Laryngeal clefts: a histopathologic study and review. Ann Otol Rhinol Laryngol 88:837–845

MacIntosh R, et al (1954) The incidence of congenital malformations: a study of 5964 pregnancies. Paediatrics 14:505–521

Petterson G (1955) Inhibited separation of larynx and the upper part of trachea from oesophagus in a newborn. Report of a case succesfully operated upon. Acta Chir Scand 10:250–255

Pracy R, Stell PM (1974) Laryngeal cleft: diagnosis and management. J Laryngol Otol 88:483–486

Richter CF (1792) Dissertatio medico de infanticido in artis obstetriciae. Thesis, Leipzig

Ruder CB, Glaser LC (1977) Anesthetic management of laryngotracheoesophageal cleft. Anesthesiology 47:65–67

Free Periosteal Grafts in Tracheal Reconstruction:

An Experimental Study

S. E. Haugen[1], T. Kufaas[1], and S. Svenningsen[1]

Introduction

In obstructive lesions of the trachea it is currently agreed that the best method of treatment is resection of the lesion followed by direct tracheal end-to-end anastomosis. On some occasions, however, this is not feasible, and recourse to other methods of reconstruction is then necessary. Various forms of grafting, with auto- and allografts, have been used both experimentally and clinically. One source of graft material, is the periosteal membrane, which is used in the form of free or pedicled grafts. It has been shown that this method leads to epithelialization of the defect, and cartilage and bone formation allows a stable tracheal wall to be obtained (Kufaas 1981; Kufaas and Pasila 1974; Olsen and Nordin 1976; Ritsilä and Alhopuro 1973).

In a previous experimental study performed in rabbits by one of us (T.K.) to clarify some of the aspects of periosteal grafting, tracheal wall defects were created operatively and immediately covered by free periosteal grafts. The conclusions after these experiments were as follows:

1. The ability of a periosteal graft to induce bone or cartilage formation when transplanted to a tracheal defect was confirmed.
2. The proliferation of the periosteal membrane seemed best when the osteogenic layer of the membrane was towards the lumen.
3. Both window and cartilaginous defects were repaired successfully.
4. Grafting with tibial periosteum resulted in more rapid healing than that with cranial periosteum (Kufaas 1981).

Present Study

In the previous experiments the grafts were applied either as patches or encircling the trachea. No patch graft gave rise to any debilitating stenosis. However, one young, growing animal with a circular graft developed a tracheal stricture. This observation induced a further experimental series to study the idea of circular periosteal grafting of the trachea in growing rabbits.

Ten rabbits 5–6 weeks old were operated upon under barbiturate anaesthesia. The trachea was dissected free through a midline cervical incision. A tracheal

---

[1]Unit of Paediatric Surgery, University Hospital, Regionsykehuset, N-7000 Trondheim, Norway.

Fig. 1. The periosteal graft in position over the tracheal defect

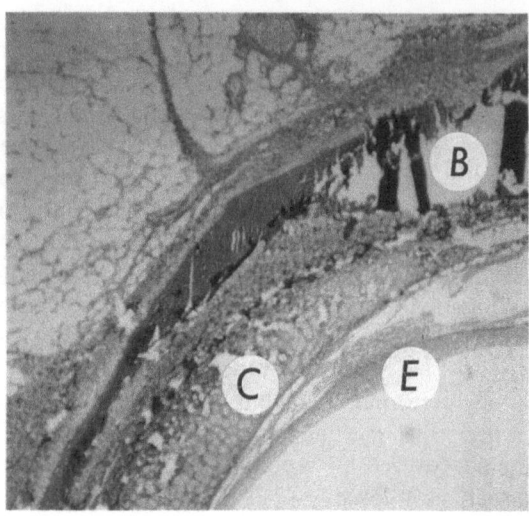

Fig. 2. Microscopic view of tracheal wall after grafting and bone formation. *B*, bone; *C*, remnant of cartilaginous ring; *E*, epithelial lining

defect was created, resecting the anterior third of three or four cartilaginous rings while leaving the mucosa intact. A strip of tibial periosteum was removed and placed in a circle around the trachea, where it was fixed in place with several sutures, covering the defect (Fig. 1). Tracheal intubation was not performed.

Two animals died 1 and 4 weeks after the operation, both with gastroenteritis. Eight rabbits lived for 3–6 months and reached full adult size, whereupon they were sacrificed. All ten tracheas were taken out and examined macro- and microscopically, with the following result: an osseous ring was present in nine cases (Fig. 2). Only in the rabbit that died after 1 week was no ossification observed. A stenosis had developed in eight animals; in six of these the stenosis was considered severe, whereas two had only slightly stenoses. One animal did not develop any stenosis.

Conclusion

After this experimental series, although small, we conclude that there is a high risk of subsequent debilitating stenosis when periosteal grafts are placed circularly over tracheal defects in rabbits.

Summary

If resection followed by end-to-end anastomosis is not possible in obstructive lesions of the trachea other methods of reconstruction must be used. The ability of a periosteal graft to induce bone or cartilage formation when transplanted to cover a tracheal defect was confirmed in a previous experimental study. In this study free tibial periosteal grafts were used for repair of tracheal defects created in rabbits. The graft was placed circumferentially around the trachea. It is concluded that there is a high risk of development of severe osseous tracheal stenosis when periosteal grafts are placed circumferentially around the trachea.

Résumé

Quand la résection et l'anastomose terminoterminale ne sont pas praticables pour la reconstitution de la trachée, il faut utiliser d'autres techniques. Une étude expérimentale préliminaire a confirmé le fait qu'un greffon périostique peut provoquer la formation d'os ou de cartilage quand il est mis en place sur une lésion de la trachée. Pour cette étude on a utilisé des greffons périostiques prélevés dans le tibia pour la reconstruction de la trachée de lapins. Le greffon a été disposé circulairement autour de la trachée. On en a conclu que le risque de provoquer una sténose osseuse grave en plaçant un greffon périostique circulaire autour de la trachée était considérable.

Zusammenfassung

Wenn eine Resektion und eine End-zu-End-Anastomose bei obstruktiven Trachealäsionen nicht möglich sind, müssen andere Rekonstruktionsmethoden zur Anwendung kommen. Die Fähigkeit periostaler Transplantate zur Bildung von Knochen oder Knorpel nach Transplantation auf Tracheadefekte wurde in einer früheren experimentellen Untersuchung bestätigt. In der vorliegenden Untersuchung wurden freie Periosttransplantate aus der Tibia zur Deckung von Tracheadefekten bei Kaninchen verwendet. Es wird der Schluß gezogen, daß nach zirkulärer Anlagerung des Transplantats um die Trachea ein hohes Risiko einer ossären Trachealstenose besteht.

References

Kufaas T (1981) Tracheal reconstruction with free periosteal grafts. An experimental study in rabbits. Scand J Thorac Cardiovasc Surg [Suppl 31]

Kufaas T, Pasila M (1974) Free periosteal transplants in tracheal reconstruction. Report on three cases. Z Kinderchir 15: 371–387

Ohlsen L, Nordin U (1976) Tracheal reconstruction with perichondrial grafts. An experimental study. Scand J Plast Reconstr Surg 10: 135–145

Ritsila V, Alhopuro S (1973) Reconstruction of experimental tracheal cartilage defects with free periosteum. A preliminary report. Scand J Plast Constr Surg 7: 116–119

Tumour-Induced Intraluminal Stenoses of the Cervical Trachea — Tumour Excision and Tracheoplasty

R. Daum[1], H. J. Denecke[2], and H. Roth[1]

Introduction

Stenoses of the subglottic or cervical trachea resulting from tumours are extremely dangerous, since they can lead rapidly to life-threatening situations as a consequence of bleeding or increasing dyspnoea. During the last 5 years, we have operated on three children with such conditions, two of whom had benign tumours and one, a sarcoma. Because of the localization and the very low incidence of tracheal tumours in childhood there is still some reserve, since such primary problems as lesions of the recurrent nerve and secondary cicatricial stenoses bring further problems in their train.

Case Histories

Case 1

This 13-year-old girl (born 5.5.1968) had presented with deepening of the voice, coughing and dyspnoea at the age of 12. A tracheal foreign body was suspected and she was admitted to an E.N.T. clinic. Tracheoscopy revealed a relatively soft, protruding tumour 20 cm down on the left side of the trachea, leaving only a fissure-like aperture at the anterior and right lateral tracheal wall. The tumour was carefully resected and bleeding was minimal. Subsequently, tracheostomy was performed. Pathohistological findings were consistent with a sarcoma not exactly identifiable. Since the initial diagnosis was rhabdomyosarcoma, combined chemo- and radiotherapy was performed. The final diagnosis indicated a sarcoma histologically not to classify but well differentiated where sensitivity of the tumor to radio- and chemotherapy could not be expected. Repeat tracheoscopy 3 months later still showed a left lateral tumour 2.5–3 cm in diameter. Both the attending doctor and father, who was himself a doctor, refused surgery since they did not expect it to be curative. The mother, however, insisted on transfer to another hospital.

First we excised the cicatricial tracheostomy scar and extended the incision down to the level of the manubrium in the midline of the trachea. There was

[1] Paediatric Surgical Department, Surgical Centre of the University of Heidelberg, Im Neuenheimer Feld 110, D-6900 Heidelberg, FRG.
[2] Hospital Speyererhof, D-6900 Heidelberg, FRG.

Progress in Pediatric Surgery, Vol. 21
Ed. by P. Wurnig
© Springer-Verlag Berlin Heidelberg 1987

thumb-nail-sized, ulcerated tumour with bulging rims at the left lateral tracheal wall. After partial resection of the trachea left laterally the remaining tracheal wall was drawn to the middle. Using magnifying glasses, we took care not to leave tumour tissue penetrating into the peritracheal connective tissue. A large skin flap originating from the anterior thoracic wall was turned in to cover the lateral tracheal defect. Since this flap did not cover the whole defect adequately a second skin flap from the left side was used to cover the defect cranially. The scars of the earlier tracheostomy were excised and the cervical skin sutured with the tracheal mucosa. An intratracheal dressing was applied and a tracheal cannula inserted; the tracheostomy hole plugged with a Miculicz tamponade.

Case 2

This baby girl, born 2.6.1978, presented with inspiratory stridor at the age of 6 weeks. She was admitted to a children's hospital with a diagnosis of false croup. Deterioration necessitated emergency tracheostomy. Laryngotracheoscopy did not definitively show a tumour. The baby was transferred to our clinic for further diagnosis and treatment. During repeat laryngotracheoscopy a subglottic narrowing was noted and suspected to be caused by an extraluminal tumour. Therefore, this region was surgically exposed, revealing an atypical lobe of the thyroid gland squeezing the trachea. The right upper pole of the thyroid gland was fixed to cervical vertebral column. The inspiratory stridor continued, however. During the further course a slight tracheal stenosis developed within the tracheostomy region owing to a mucosal fold, which was resected. A further tracheoscopy revealed a well-rounded, elastic tumour below the glottis on the right side, impairing the passage of air. The trachea was opened in the midline above the tracheostomy and below the thyroid cartilage. There was a sessile, smooth tumour narrowing the tracheal lumen. The mucosa was carefully incised and the tumour was removed step by step. A skin flap was fixed to the tracheal rims in the usual manner, i.e. primary closure of the trachea was not performed. Pathohistological findings were first interpreted as indicative of dystopic thyroid tissue. Serial sections, however, led to the diagnosis of a haemangioma. There was a perfect mucosal lining of the trachea 6 weeks after surgery. The tracheal cannula was withdrawn 3 weeks later. The last follow-up was performed 6 months after surgery, showing free passage of air and a normal voice.

Case 3

Only a few days after birth, 20.2.1980, this neonate was observed to have progressive respiratory distress. He was admitted to our hospital at the age of 4 months. The findings at laryngotracheoscopy, however, were normal. Considerable dyspnoea necessitated tracheostomy with skin plasty according to Denecke. Repeat laryngotracheoscopy 8 months later revealed a subglottic tumour directly below the cricoid on the right side, narrowing the lumen considerably. Under intubation anaesthesia the cricoid was incised and the tumour submucosally removed from the lateral and posterior tracheal wall. A skin flap was sutured with the conoid

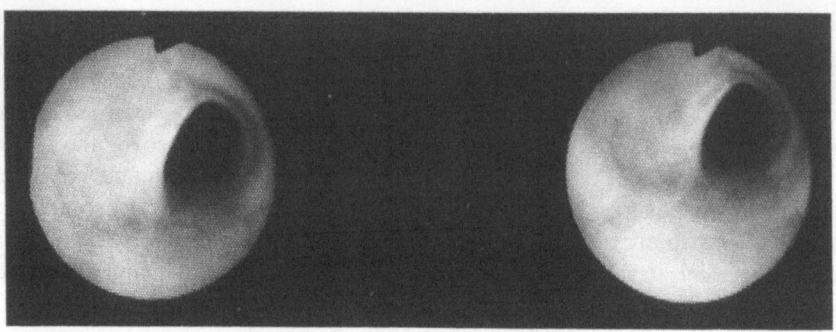

Fig. 1. Status after partial resection of the trachea for sarcoma. Tracheoscopy 2¼ years after surgery. Note the clearly recognizable skin flap inserted

ligament, and a Mikulicz tamponade and a tracheal cannula were inserted. Pathohistological examination revealed a haemangioma. Retrograde laryngoscopy 3 months later showed good laryngeal dynamics. The voice was normal and no stenosis was evident. Follow-up endoscopy another 2 months later did not reveal tumour recurrence and showed normal laryngeal function. The child was decannulated and the tracheostomy hole covered with skin; the inner region was not closed, to avoid stridor. Follow-up 7 months after surgery showed normal conditions.

Clinical Symptoms

Clinical symptoms depend on the site and size of the tumour. Minor tumours may remain undetected for some years, since the trachea can be narrowed by one third of its lumen without producing any symptoms. Our patients, however, presented with symptoms at times ranging from right after birth up to 6 weeks after birth, leading to the differential diagnosis of a vascular ring in various forms and extratracheal tumours such as duplications or congenital struma. Symptoms can change suddenly in the case of pediculated haemangiomas effecting subtotal airways obstruction. In older children a pathological process in the cervical trachea may change the voice, as was the case in our 13-year-old patient with sarcoma.

Diagnosis

A plain cervical X-ray in the lateral position should be taken first, to exclude tracheal displacement. Oesophageal contrast radiography discloses the relations between oesophagus, trachea and vertebral column. A-P X-rays allow differentiation between intra- and extraluminal processes. Tomography of the cervical trachea is difficult in small children, and of limited significance with minor intraluminal tumours. A CT scan, or even more likely, an NMR scan may allow diagnosis.

It is self-evident that endotracheal examination is of great importance, since modern instruments allow an accurate diagnosis even in small children. Only in the subglottic region can small tumours be missed. There is no experience with lung function tests in children to specify the site and extent of an airways obstruction, since small children do not cooperate.

Treatment

The treatment of choice is surgical removal of the tumour, since irradiation of a haemangioma, for instance, may induce additional complications, such as local stenosis or malignant degeneration of the thyroid gland after a latency period of 15–20 years. Various surgical methods are possible, depending on the site and histological status of the tumour and the age of the patient.

Endoscopical resection
Complete resection of the trachea
Partial resection of the trachea with plastic reconstruction

Endoscopical resection is highly problematic in small infants, because everything is so small. Complete resection is indicated if the tumour is located in the middle segment of the cervical trachea. There is an increasing danger of recurrent nerve lesions if the tumour is located directly in the subglottic area. Moreover, the voice becomes deeper and remains so permanently as a consequence of manipulation of the cricoid.

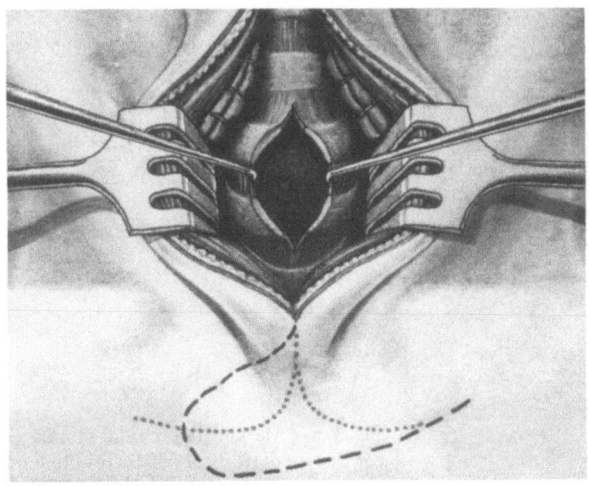

Fig. 2. Plastic tracheostomy. The skin flaps to be turned in are marked to avoid vascular erosions

We therefore prefer the method published by Denecke, which is the least stressful for patient and surgeon. It is performed in stages, a tracheal cleft being left after partial resection in the first session. In a second session the tracheal cleft is closed by plastic surgery.

Operative Procedure

First a plastic tracheostomy is performed, during which pediculated skin flaps are sutured with the tracheal rims (Fig. 2). With this method there are practically no vascular erosions. For tumour removal the trachea is opened in the midline and,

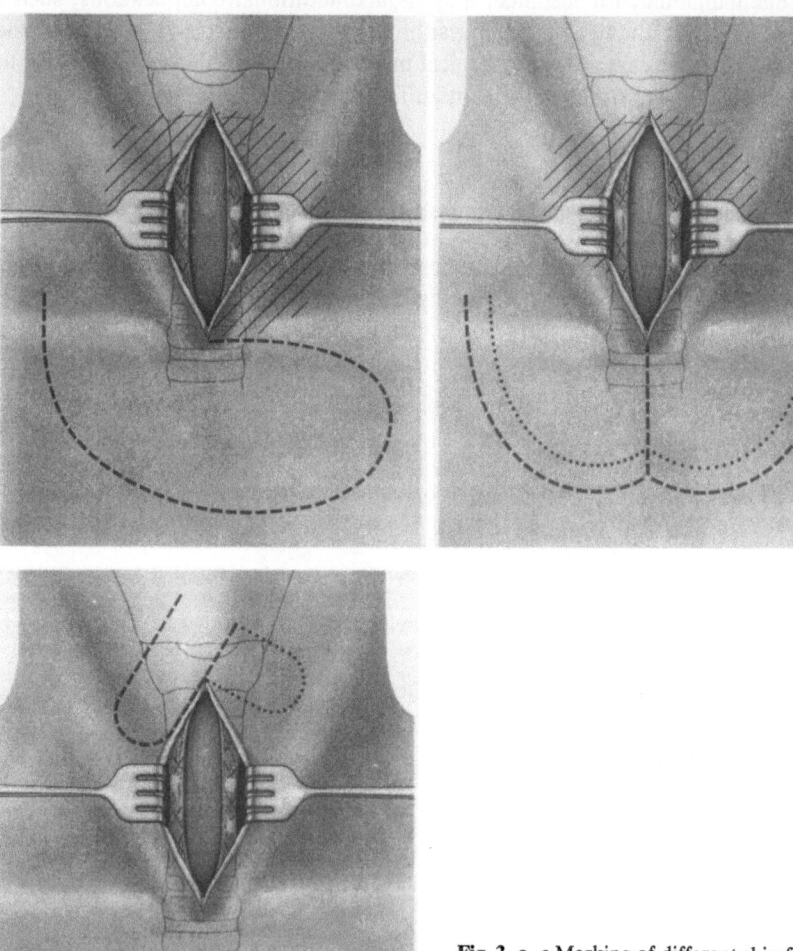

Fig. 3. a–c Marking of different skin flaps for closure of tracheal defects resulting from tumour resection (from Denecke 1980)

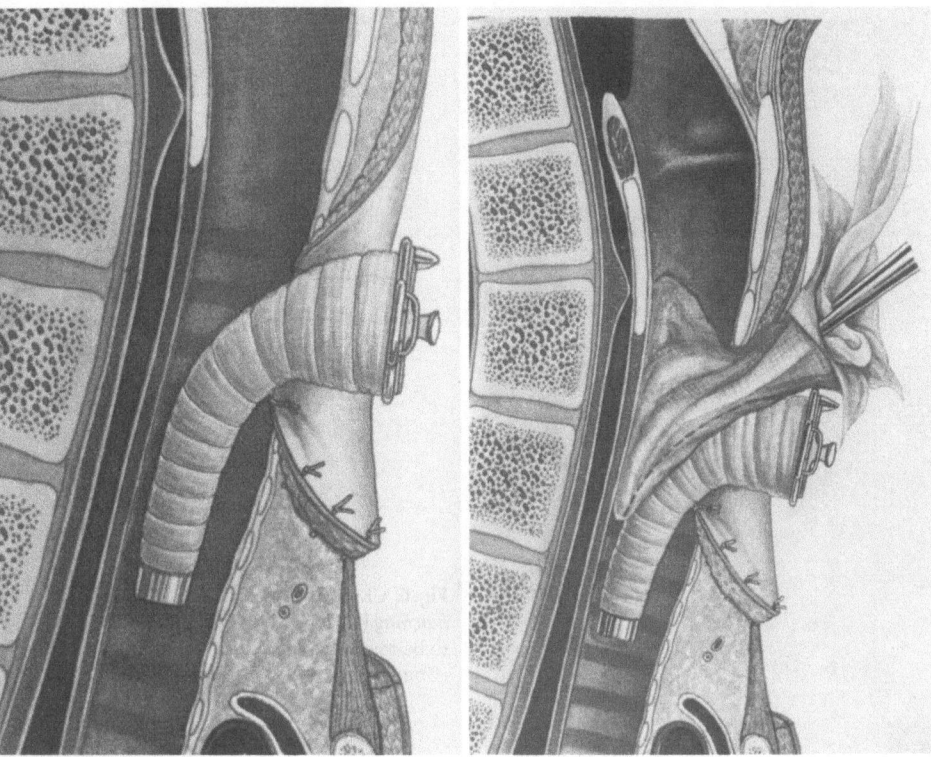

5

Fig. 4. Lateral view of the turned-in skin flap and the tracheal cannula taped in place with gauze (from Denecke 1980)

Fig. 5. Additional plugging with a Mikulicz tamponade (from Denecke 1980)

depending on the findings, in the case of a haemangioma the tumour is either resected together with the mucosa or a partial resection of the trachea performed. In every case the trachea is joined with skin after mobilization of a skin flap resulting in an open tracheal cleft (Fig. 3). A tracheal cannula taped with gauze is inserted into this cleft (Fig. 4). In addition, the cleft is plugged with Mikulicz tamponade, thus avoiding the flow of secretions into the bronchial tree (Fig. 5). The tamponade is changed every 3–4 days. After temporary closure of the cleft with adhesive plaster the cleft is peritomised and closed in the craniocaudal direction 6–8 weeks later (Fig. 6). If there is too much tension on the suture a Z-plasty can be carried out.

The maintenance of the tracheal cleft after the first session has the great advantage that complete tracheal resection can be avoided in many instances. The method can be applied not only in tracheal tumours but also in congenital and acquired stenoses and for establishment of tracheostomies. This means that the complication rate is minimal.

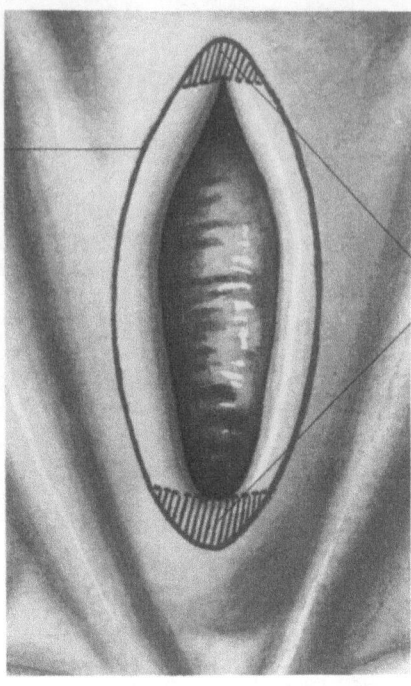

Fig. 6. Closure of tracheal cleft. *Cross-hatching* indicates areas of skin that may need to be removed. *Heavy line* indicates incision (from Denecke 1980)

Summary

Three children with stenoses of the cervical trachea caused by tumours are reported on.

The first was a 13-year-old girl with a sarcoma of the tracheal wall 20 cm down. We performed partial resection of the trachea and turned a skin flap according to Denecke into the defect.

In the second case a capillary haemangioma had caused severe stenosis, requiring resection of the tumour together with the tracheal mucosa. A haemangioma had caused tracheal stenosis in the third case, too; in this child partial tracheal resection and skin flap plasty were performed. The postoperative course was uneventful in all three children. So far, there is no recurrence of the sarcoma 4½ years after operation.

Résumé

Trois cas d'enfants présentant une sténose de la trachée cervicale, due une tumeur, ont été observés.

Dans le premier cas, il s'agit d'une jeune fille de 13 ans avec un sarcome de la paroi de la trachée, à une profondeur d'une vingtaine de cm. Nous avons procédé

Cardiopulmonary Bypass in Tracheal Surgery in Infants and Small Children

I. Louhimo[1] and M. Leijala[1]

Introduction

Mild and moderate tracheal stenosis can be effectively treated by various intra-bronchial procedures. Severe stenosis with almost total obstruction of the trachea is best managed by tracheal resection, which is a safe and established procedure in adults and older children. Problems arise when a small child has severe stenosis of the distal trachea, where tracheostomy is of no help. Only ten cases of successful resection of thoracic trachea in infants have been described (de Beaujeu and Louis 1984; Debrand et al. 1979; Mansfield 1980; Salzer et al. 1985; Weber et al. 1982). In these patients ventilation during the operation was carried out through an endotracheal tube in one or two of the bronchi. As already reported (Louhimo and Leijala 1985), we have used cardiopulmonary bypass on five occasions for distal tracheal resection in infants under 2 years of age. We believe it is the method of choice in the treatment of this difficult problem.

Patients and Method

Patients

The overall experience in the treatment of tracheal stenosis at the Children's Hospital, University of Helsinki, has been described in earlier papers (Kufaas and Pasila 1974; Louhimo and Leijala 1985; Louhimo et al. 1971). Two patients, aged 8 and 9 years, had successful tracheal resection with cardiopulmonary bypass in 1966. In 1970–1972 plastic operations on the distal trachea were performed with bypass in two patients, aged 10 and 27 months. They both eventually died. In this connection only the technical aspects of distal tracheal resection in patients under 2 years of age are discussed. Four such patients were operated on, their ages at operation being 6 weeks, 7 months, 16 months and 21 months. The last patient had a second resection at the age of 24 months.

[1]Department of Paediatric Surgery, Children's Hospital, Helsinki University Central Hospital, Stenbäckinkatu 11, SF-00290 Helsinki 29, Finnland.

Progress in Pediatric Surgery, Vol. 21
Ed. by P. Wurnig
© Springer-Verlag Berlin Heidelberg 1987

à une résection partielle de la trachée et mis en place un lambeau cutané de rotation selon Denecke.

Dans le second cas, un hémangiome capillaire était à l'origine d'unse sténose grave qui nous obligea à pratiquer une résection de la tumeur et de la muqueuse trachéale. Dans le troisième cas, il s'agissait également d'un hémangiome à l'origine d'une sténose de la trachée. Une résection fut pratiquée et un lambeau cutané fut utilisé pour la reconstitution. L'évolution post-opératoire fut satisfaisante dans les trois cas. Jusqu'à présent, 4 ans et demi aprés l'intervention, il n'y a pas eu récidive du sarcome.

Zusammenfassung

Es wird über 3 Kinder mit intraluminalen tumorbedingten Stenosen der zervikalen Trachea berichtet.

Im ersten Fall handelte es sich um ein 13jähriges Mädchen mit einem Sarkom, das in 19–20 cm Tiefe an der linken Trachealwand gelegen war. Es wurde eine Trachealteilresektion durchgeführt und ein Hautschwenklappen nach Denecke in den Defekt eingeschlagen. Im zweiten Fall führte ein kapilläres Hämangiom zu einer erheblichen Stenose. Der Tumor wurde stückchenweise mit der Schleimhaut entfernt.

Im dritten Fall war ebenfalls ein Hämangiom Ursache der Stenose. Nach Teilresektion wurde ebenfalls eine Hautschiebelappenplastik vorgenommen. Der postoperative Verlauf war bei allen Kindern unauffällig. Ein Rezidiv des Sarkoms ist bisher, 4½ Jahre nach dem Eingriff, nicht aufgetreten.

Reference

Denecke HJ (1980) Die oto-rhino-laryngologischen Operationen im Mund- und Halsbereich. Springer, Berlin Heidelberg New York

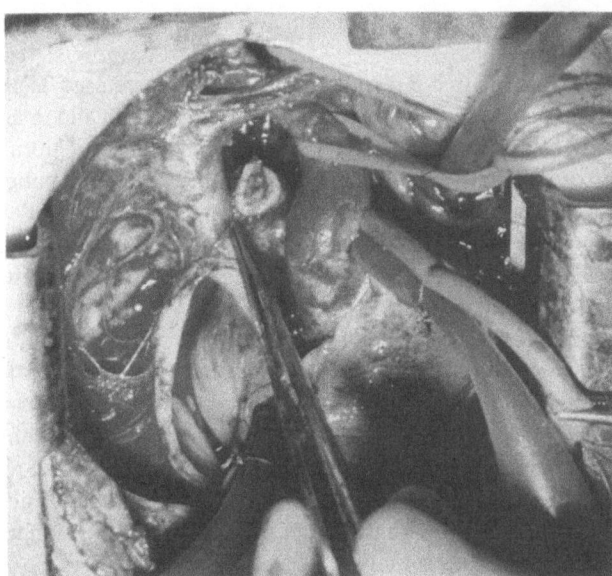

Fig. 1. Peroperative view of tracheal resection through median sternotomy with cardiopulmonary bypass. The aorta and right atrium are cannulated. The distal end of the divided and almost completely abstructed trachea is seen just above the forceps

Operative Approach

A skin incision is made from the jugulum to the xiphoid process and the sternum divided longitudinally as in routine preparation for cardiac-surgery. The superior vena cava is dissected free from its entry into the right atrium to its branching. The innominate vein is lifted upwards. The right pulmonary artery and the aorta and the innominate artery are also freed. The trachea is situated between the superior vena cava and the aorta to right and left and between the innominate vein and right pulmonary artery above and below (Fig. 1). The lymphatic tissue present in the front of the trachea and below the carina is removed, and in this way the lower half of the trachea and both bronchi can be exposed and dissected free. If there is previous tracheostomy and a long resection is expected the tracheostomy site must be mobilized to prevent tension on the anastomosis.

Once the trachea is dissected free, the pericardium is opened and the patient is heparinized. The ascending aorta is cannulated and a single venous cannula is introduced into the right atrium through the atrial appendix. A normothermic partial cardiopulmonary bypass is started without closing the aorta or the caval veins. Respiration is stopped and the trachea divided at the site of the most severe stenosis, which, however, cannot be seen from outside. Slices of trachea upwards and downwards are then cut away until a normal tracheal lumen is found. From this approach it is possible to remove the whole distal half of the trachea, and if necessary also the main bronchi. In one of our cases the upper right lobe was also removed during this dissection and an anastomosis made between the right intermediate bronchus and lower trachea.

The tracheal anastomosis is secured interrupted sutures. We have used Ticron in three cases, Prolene in one case and PDS in one case. Theoretically and in animal experiments, absorbable suture material allows a better chance of normal tracheal growth afterwards. While the anastomosis is made the neck of the patient is bent forwards and kept in this position by pillows or a premade plaster-of-Paris cast. When the anastomosis is ready, its air leakage is tested under water. The perfusion is then stopped, the heart decannulated, and the operation ended after routine haemostasis and mediastinal drainage.

During the postoperative period our patients have been kept relaxed with nondepolarizing muscle relaxants and ventilated mechanically. The necessity for these procedures cannot be confirmed. They were instituted firstly to prevent any sudden movement of the neck and diaphragm and secondly to provide easy ventilation with constantly low airwaypressure. In addition the neck of the patient was kept flexed by using a preoperatively made plaster of Paris cast on three occasion, and by supporting the head with a pillow on two other occasions. The position was maintained for one to two weeks after surgery.

Results

The 6-week-old baby in whom resection of the lower part of the trachea, the upper right lobe of the lung and both bronchi was performed died on the day after the operation. In this infant it was not possible to find any bronchial lumen of normal caliber, and this led to too narrow an anastomosis. In the oldest child the primary resection of 1.5 cm of precarinal trachea was too limited and resulted in restenosis above the anastomosis. Two and half months after the first procedure a second resection of 2.5 cm of the trachea was performed, and after that the child recovered. In the 7-month-old and 16-month-old babies resection was uneventful. The follow-up time of the three living patients is now 3–5 years.

The use of cardiopulmonary bypass and heparinization of the patients have produced no problems. Cardiopulmonary bypass makes the resection both unhurried and easy. In two patients with most severe stenosis the help of bypass was necessary even during dissection of the trachea, because oxygenation was otherwise difficult.

Discussion

Tracheal resections are now usually performed without the use of extracorporeal circulation. If the stenosis is very narrow and ventilation difficult forceful dilatation with an endoscope or endotracheal tube is recommended to maintain a patent airway during anaesthetic induction (Grillo 1973). This procedure, however, is not without risk, and we and others have caused tracheal rupture under such circumstances.

The group with most experience of infant tracheal resections (Nakayama et al. 1982) has stated that they have not found cardiopulmonary bypass necessary. Nonetheless, one of their patients died of asphyxia on the table, and one of de Beaujeu's patients (de Beaujeu et al. 1984) had a cardiac arrest during the operation. These findings, together with our own experience of the ease of cardiopulmonary bypass, make us believe it is the safest way of providing good operative conditions in a small infant needing resection of the carinal area. The provision of a standby heart-lung machine is not adequate, because sudden respiratory failure may not allow enough time for commencement of the perfusion.

Of course, the use of perfusion in infants and small children is safe only it is routinely practised for paediatric cardiac surgery. In the early 1970s, when we operated on two young patients with tracheal problems, certain difficulties resulted from the perfusion itself. At that time perfusions in infancy were rare. Today most of the open heart surgery at our hospital is performed in patients under the age of 2 years. Accordingly perfusions have caused no problems in our recent patients. Partial perfusion with beating heart was sufficient for oxygenation. The perfusion cannulae were not in the way; on the contrary, they make aortic and pulmonary artery distortion easier and safer. No tubes are present in bronchi, which makes operation easy. There is no need for hurried surgery. Similar opinions have been expressed by Idriss et al. (1984) with reference to pericardial patch tracheoplasties in five infants.

Medial sternotomy with cervical extension, if needed, gives an excellent approach to the whole trachea and main bronchi, irrespective of the length of the trachea. In the first resection patient in 1966 the right thoracotomy approach was used, but it was not as easy as the median sternotomy from the bypass point of view, and the femoral artery had to be used for cannulation. The 6-week-old baby died because healthy tissue in the distal bronchi was not present in sufficient amounts to provide a patent airway; there were no problems with perfusion or other technical difficulties.

Postoperative care has been somewhat improvised, as there was no information available on infant tracheal surgery in 1980 when we started. We do not know whether postoperative curarization is necessary in these patients, but we have so far used it for safety reasons. Nakayama et al. (1982) recommend a forward position of the neck for 6 weeks, but we have used it only for 2 weeks. This appeared to be sufficient even in patients in whom one half of the trachea was resected. Postoperative management in the intensive care unit is often prolonged, and emergency bronchoscopy facilities must be available at all times.

A warning is given about bronchoscopy and dilatation of severe distal tracheal stenosis. Even a simple bronchoscopic examination produced severe difficulties in all our cases, and made surgery necessary as a matter of some urgency in one patient. The same opinion has been expressed by other authors (Idriss et al. 1984; Mansfield 1980; Nakayama et al. 1982). Accordingly, endobronchial procedures, including laser treatment, are potentially very dangerous manoeuvers in distal stenosis and may lead to the death of the patient. The best treatment for severe restenosis seems to be a repeat resection, and not endobronchial manipulation.

Tracheoplasty with cartilage or pericardium is another alternative if the stenosis is not extreme (Idriss et al. 1984; Meyer 1983). Distal tracheal stenosis in infancy remains a difficult problem. The use of modern methods of cardiopulmonary bypass gives a useful extra means of successful treatment.

Summary

Five resections of the distal trachea with cardiopulmonary bypass were carried out in four children aged 6 weeks to 24 months. Only technical aspects are discussed, and the operative method is described in detail. The use of cardiopulmonary bypass and heparinization of the patients did not cause any problmes. Cardiopulmonary bypass allows an easy and unhurried procedure. Although other authors do not regard cardiopulmonary bypass as necessary in similar circumstances, we believe that it is the safest way of providing optimal operative conditions and results in surgery of distal tracheal stenoses.

Résumé

Cinq résections de la trachée distale avec bypass cardiopulmonaire ont été pratiquées dans le cas de quatre enfants âgés de 6 mois à deux ans. Il n'est question ici que des aspects techniques et la méthode d'intervention est décrite en détails. Le bypass cardiopulmonaire et l'héparinisation des patients n'ont causé aucun problème. Le bypass cardiopulmonaire permet une intervention facile et sans hâte. Bien que d'autres auteurs soient d'avis que le bypass cardiopulmonaire ne soit pas nécessaire dans ce genre d'intervention, nous trouvons qu'il constitue le moyen le plus sûr pour effectuer l'intervention dans les meilleures conditions possibles ct obtenir les résultats voulus.

Zusammenfassung

Fünf Resektionen der distalen Trachea wurden unter kardiopulmonalem Bypass an 4 Kindern im Alter von 6 Wochen bis 24 Monaten durchgeführt. Es werden nur technische Aspekte diskutiert und die Operationstechnik ist im Detail beschrieben. Die Verwendung des kardiopulmonalen Bypasses und der Heparinisierung der Patienten verursachte keinerlei Probleme. Der kardiopulmonale Bypass ermöglicht ein einfaches Verfahren ohne Eile. Obwohl andere Autoren den kardiopulmonalen Bypass unter ähnlichen Umständen nicht für erforderlich halten, sind wir der Ansicht, daß dieser am sichersten optimale Operationsbedingungen und Resultate in der Chirurgie distaler Trachealstenosen gewährleistet.

References

De Beaujeu MJ, Louis D (1984) Obstruction par sténoses trachéales et bronchiques congénitales. Chir Pediatr 25:249–260

Debrand M, Tsueda K, Browning SK, et al (1979) Anesthesia for extensive resection of congenital tracheal stenosis in an infant. Anesth Analg 58:431–433

Grillo HC (1973) Reconstruction of the trachea. Experience in 100 consecutive cases. Thorax 28: 667–679

Idriss FS, DeLeon SY, Ilbawi MN, et al (1984) Tracheoplasty with pericardial patch for extensive tracheal stenosis in infants and children. J Thorac Cardiovasc Surg 88:527–536

Kufaas T, Pasila M (1974) Free periosteal transplants in tracheal reconstruction. Z Kinderchir 15:371–387

Louhimo I, Leijala M (1985) The treatment of low retrosternal tracheal stenosis in the neonate and small children. Thorac Cardiovasc Surg 33:98–102

Louhimo I, Grahne B, Pasila M, Suutarinen T (1971) Acquired laryngotracheal stenosis in children. J Pediatr Surg 6:730–737

Mansfield P (1980) Tracheal resection in infancy. J Pediatr Surg 15:79–81

Meyer R (1983) Reconstructive surgery of the trachea. Thieme, Stuttgart

Nakayama DK, Harrison MR, de Lorimer AA, et al (1982) Reconstructive surgery for obstructing lesions of the intrathoracic trachea in infants and small children. J Pediatr Surg 17:854–868

Salzer GM, Hartl H, Wurnig P (1985) Resektionsbehandlung bei Trachealstenosen im frühen Kindesalter. Paper presented at the 14th International Symposium of the Österreichische Gesellschaft für Kinderchirurgie, Obergurgl, January 28–30, 1985

Weber TR, Eigen H, Scott PH, et al (1982) Resection of congenital tracheal stenosis involving the carina. J Thorac Cardiovasc Surg 84:200–203

Resection of an Intrathoracic Tracheal Stenosis in a Child

T. A. Angerpointner[1], W. Stelter[2], K. Mantel[1], and W. Ch. Hecker[1]

Introduction

Prolonged endotracheal intubation and congenital malformations are the most common causes of distal narrowing of the trachea in infancy and childhood (Mansfield 1980; O'Neill 1984). Resection of the stenosis with subsequent end-to-end anastomosis has proved to be the treatment of choice in older patients (Grillo 1976) and was first successfully performed in the paediatric age group by Carcassonne et al. (1973). We report on a case with postintubational distal tracheal stenosis where resection of one-third of the trachea and subsequent primary anastomosis were successfully performed.

Case Report

A 6-year-old boy sustained a severe head injury during a traffic accident. A CT scan revealed right frontal and left temporal contusion haemorrhages. The patient had to be intubated for 3 days.

Rapid neurological improvement was followed by steadily increasing dyspnoea and inspiratory stridor 2 weeks later. The patient developed severe tracheal stenosis within 4 weeks after extubation and was then intubated and transferred to our hospital by helicopter as an emergency.

Emergency tracheoscopy revealed a pulsating, concentric, intrathoracic tracheal stenosis with a residual lumen 3 mm in diameter, starting 3.7 cm below the cricoid and extending over 2.3 cm, to end 3 cm above the carina. First, the stenosis was dilated and splinted with a 6-mm Vygon endotracheal tube. The boy made a good recovery, breathing spontaneously while the tube remained in place. However, when the tube was removed for tracheoscopy the stenotic area demonstrably collapsed and caused an obstruction again. Oesophageal radiography and angiography excluded an oesophageal or vascular origin of the tracheal stenosis.

We performed the operation on 29 February, 1984, 12 days after referral and 6 weeks after the accident. A Kocher collar incision was made, and the entire

[1]Paediatric Surgical Clinic, Dr. von Haunersches Kinderspital of the University of Munich, Lindwurmstraße 4, D-8000 Munich, FRG.
[2]Surgical Hospital of the University of Munich, Klinikum Großhadern, Marchioninistraße 15, D-8000 Munich 70, FRG.

Figs. 1–11. *Procedure adopted for resection of intrathoracic tracheal stenosis*

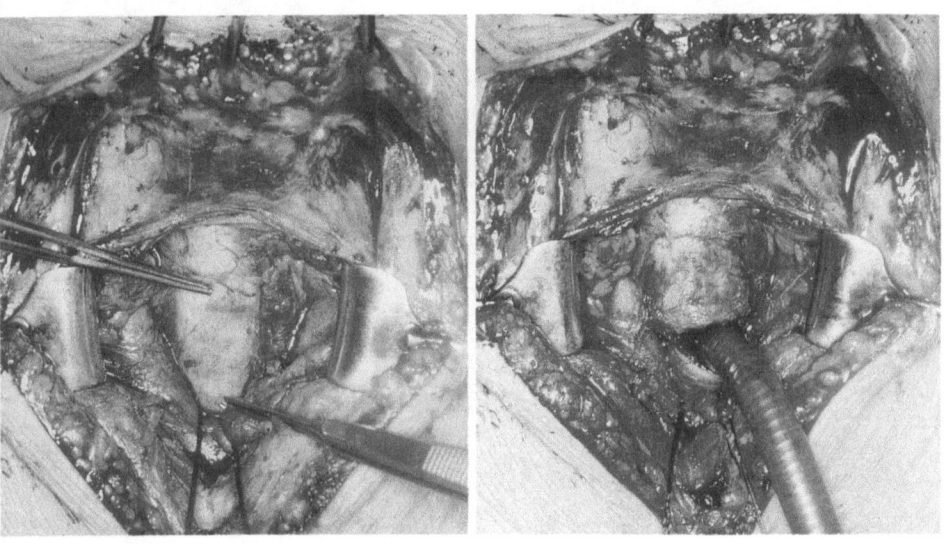

Fig. 1. Exposure of intrathoracic tracheal stenosis by way of a Kocher collar incision. The two forceps indicate the extent of the stenosis

Fig. 2. Anterior tracheal wall opened below the stenosis and lower trachea intubated with a stiff endotracheal tube. Note holding sutures in the lower tracheal segment

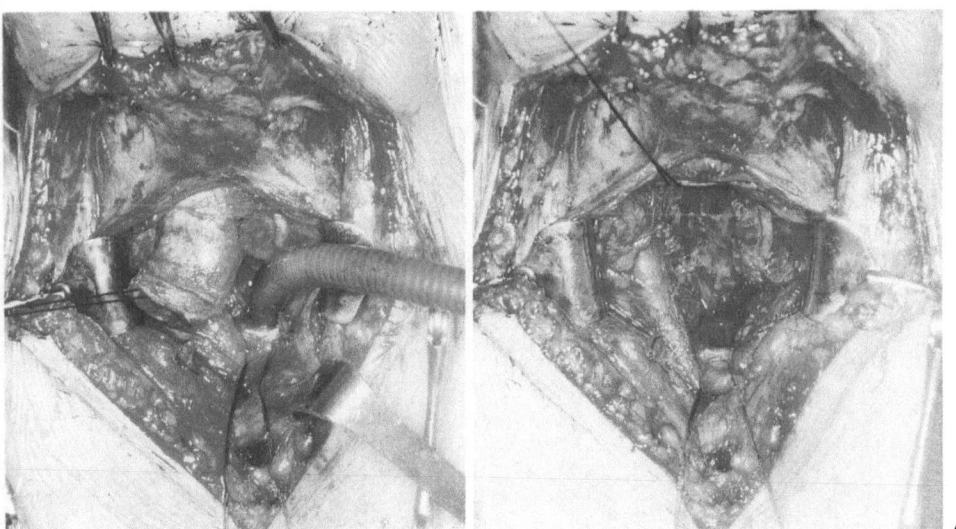

Fig. 3. Lower resection plane

Fig. 4. Upper and lower resection planes following resection of a 3-cm segment of the trachea. Note holding sutures in upper and lower segments. Endotracheal tube has been removed for a second to show extent of the stenosis

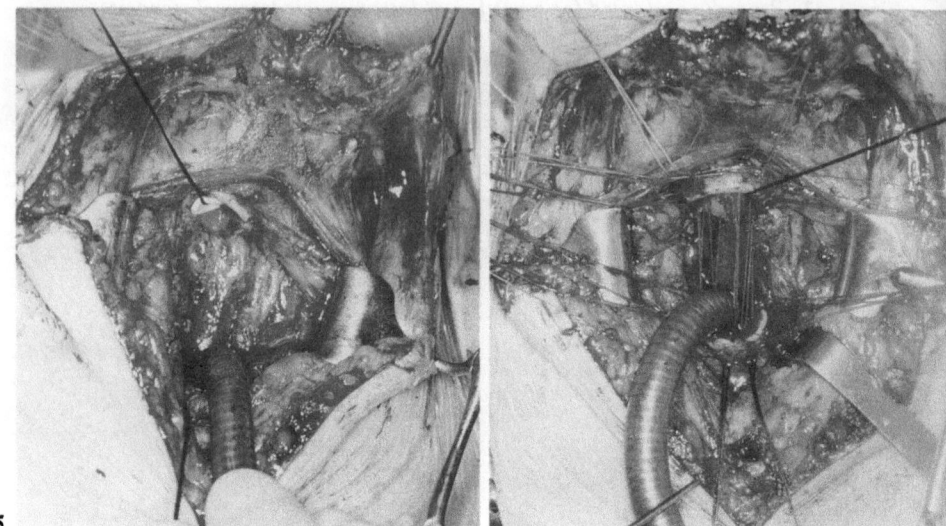

5

Fig. 5. Endotracheal tube in place again

Fig. 6. After mobilization of the tracheal segments the 4-0 Dexon interrupted sutures are already in place, but not yet tied

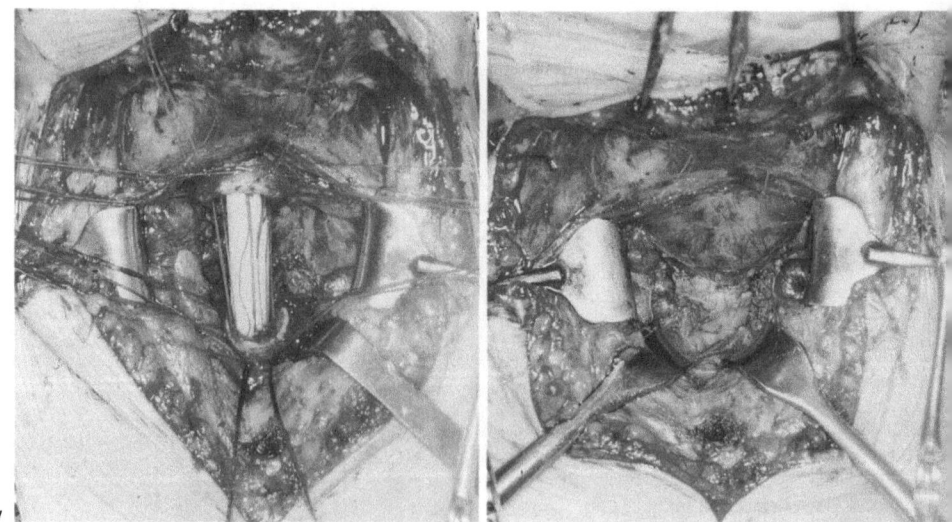

7

Fig. 7. Stiff endotracheal tube has been replaced by tube advanced over the tracheal gap

Fig. 8. Anastomosis completed

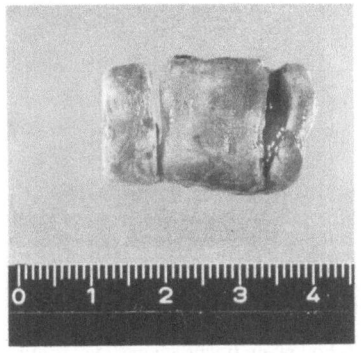

Fig. 9. Resected specimen (3 cm)

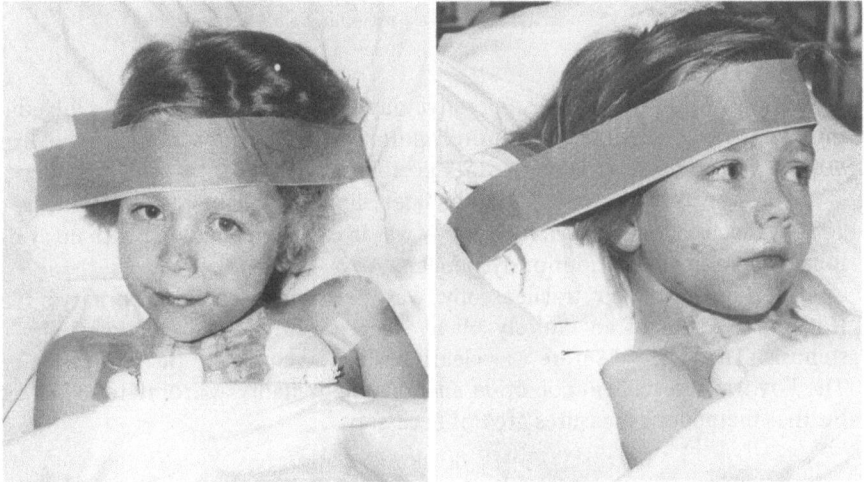

10

11

Figs. 10, 11. Two views of patient to illustrate postoperative posture of the head, fixed in cervical flexion to prevent tension on the anastomosis

stenotic region was resected within a 3-cm segment of the trachea; tracheal continuity was restored by means of 2-0 Dexon interrupted sutures, using the technique described by Grillo in 1965. Figures 1–11 illustrate the course of the operation. The resected 3 cm corresponded to 33% of the total length of the trachea (9 cm).

The boy was extubated while still in the operating room. Pathohistological findings were consistent with an unspecific, superficially ulcerous, chronically granulating and cicatricial inflammation with regenerative squamous epithelial metaplasia and without cell atypia.

Postoperatively, the head was maintained in a flexed position for 2 weeks to prevent tension on the anastomosis. Ultrasonic nebulization of Karlsbad salt was applied, and the postoperative course was entirely uneventful. The skin sutures

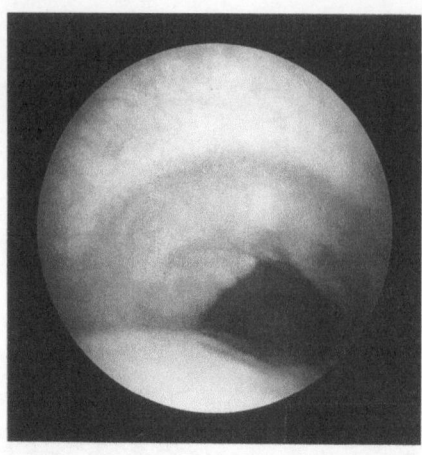

Fig. 12. Follow-up tracheoscopy 2 years after tracheal resection. Entirely bland trachea with no signs of instability or stenosis. Anastomotic region is clearly recognizable

were removed on the 9th postoperative day. The neurological status, including the electroencephalogram, was entirely normalized. The boy was discharged from hospital in good condition on the 15th postoperative day.

Follow-up tracheoscopy 3 months later showed a slight residual stenosis of 20% in the anastomotic region. The boy was in excellent condition with no symptoms and no signs of stridor or dyspnoea.

The last follow-up tracheoscopy was performed on 14 February, 1986 (Fig. 12). We found an entirely bland trachea with no signs of instability or stenosis. The tracheal suture was clearly visible 2 years after tracheal resection. The boy was in excellent condition and exhibited vitality appropriate to his age. Further therapeutic measures are not necessary.

Discussion

Dilatation or endoscopic resection of distal tracheal stenoses are often of transient success only (Heberer et al. 1980). Since the introduction of circumferential resection and reconstruction of the mediastinal or cervical trachea by Grillo in 1965, more than 700 cases have been reported in adults (Halsband and Valesky 1985). Whereas 2–4 cm was formerly regarded as the maximum length it was possible to resect, up to 70% of the adult trachea, i.e. 7–8 cm, may now be resected, since tension on the anastomosis can be reduced by several methods of mobilization, such as laryngeal mobilization and dissection of the lung hilus (Schildberg et al. 1980a, b). Successful resection of a piece of trachea as long as 7.4 cm was carried out an 24 September 1979 by W. J. Stelter (reported by Heberer et al. 1980), with an excellent result maintained up to the present.

However, circumferential resection of distal tracheal stenoses was not performed in the paediatric age group until 1973 (Caracassonne et al. 1973) because of concern about subsequent tracheal growth (Mansfield 1980). Maeda and Grillo

(1973) showed that tracheal anastomoses in puppies grew almost normally, resulting in only 20% narrowing of the lumen in the adult dog. (We have also found a slight residual stenosis of 20% in our patient.)

Since the work of Maeda and Grillo (1973), tracheal resection has been performed even in neonates and small children (Harrison et al. 1980; Nakayama et al. 1982). The maximum length resected was 2.7 cm hitherto, whereas 3 cm of the trachea (33%) was resected in our case.

We agree with other authors (Harrison et al. 1980; Nakayama et al. 1982) that it is very important to maintain the head and neck in a flexed position after the operation, to reduce tension on the anastomosis. Searching through the literature, Halsband and Valesky (1985) found only 27 cases of tracheal resection in the paediatric age group. When the cases reported at the 14th International Symposium on Tracheal and Lung Surgery in Infancy and Childhood in Obergurgl/ Austria, January 1985, were added, this number increased to 41 cases. At this meeting two cases of resection of the tracheobronchial bifurcation were presented. One was performed with the aid of cardiopulmonary bypass (Louhimo and Leijala 1985), and the other without (Salzer et al. 1985). Good to excellent results were reported by all authors who performed circumferential resection and subsequent primary anastomosis for distal tracheal stenosis in infancy and childhood. Therefore, this kind of treatment should be preferred to the plastic and reconstructive methods formerly in use.

Summary

A 6-year-old boy sustained a severe head injury during a traffic accident. He was first treated at another hospital. Despite a short intubation period of only 3 days, within 4 weeks he developed severe tracheal stenosis, with a residual lumen 3 mm in diameter and a total length of 2.3 cm, ending 3 cm above the carina. After initial bougienage enlarging the lumen to 6 mm in diameter, surgery was performed at our hospital 6 weeks after the accident. The stenosis was resected in toto, and tracheal continuity was restored by interrupted sutures using the Grillo technique. The postoperative course was uneventful. Follow-up tracheoscopy 3 months later showed a residual stenosis of 20% within the anastomotic region, and the patient was free of symptoms.

Résumé

Un petit garçon de 6 ans présentait une lésion cranioencéphalique grave après un accident de la route. Il fut d'abord traité dans un autre hôpital. En dépit d'une durée d'intubation assez courte, 3 jours seulement, il présenta en l'espace d'un mois une sténose trachéale grave avec lumière de 3 mm de diamètre seulement sur une longueur totale de 2.3 cm. La sténose se terminait à 3 cm au dessus de la carène. Nous avons d'abord dilaté la lumière avec une bougie et obtenu 6 mm de diamètre puis nous avons pratiqué l'intervention 6 semaines après l'accident: résection de la sténose et rétablissement de la continuité trachéale par sutures à points séparés selon la méthode de Grillo. L'évolution post-opératoire fut satisfaisante. Une trachéoscopie, pratiquée 3 mois après l'intervention, indiqua une sténose résiduelle de 20% au niveau de l'anastomose. Le patient ne présentait plus aucun trouble.

Zusammenfassung

Ein 6jähriger Junge erlitt bei einem Verkehrsunfall ein schweres Schädel-Hirn-Trauma, das in einer auswärtigen Klinik behandelt wurde. Trotz einer Intubationszeit von nur 3 Tagen entwickelte er innerhalb von 4 Wochen eine schwere Trachealstenose mit einem Restlumen von 3 mm im Durchmesser und einer Länge von 2,3–3 cm oberhalb der Carina. Nach anfänglicher Aufbougierung mit einem 6-mm-Tubus wurde die Operation 6 Wochen nach dem Unfall durchgeführt. Dabei wurde die Stenose in ganzer Länge von 3 cm reseziert und die Kontinuität der Trachea End-zu-End mit Einzelknopfnähten nach der Grillo-Technik wiederhergestellt. Der postoperative Verlauf war komplikationslos. Die Kontroll-Tracheoskopie 3 Monate nach der Operation ergab bei klinischer Beschwerdefreiheit des Patienten noch eine geringgradige Reststenose von 20% im Anastomosenbereich.

References

Carcassonne M, Dor V, Aubert J (1973) Tracheal resection with primary anastomosis in children. J Pediatr Surg 8:1

Grillo HC (1965) Circumferential resection and reconstruction of the mediastinal and cervical trachea. Ann Surg 162:374

Grillo HC (1976) Congenital lesions, neoplasms and injuries of the trachea. In: Sabiston DC, Spencer FC (eds) Gibbon's surgery of the chest, 3rd edn. Saunders, Philadelphia

Halsband H, Valesky A (1985) Langstreckige Trachea-Kontinuitäts-Resektion im frühen Kindesalter. Paper presented at the 14th International Symposium: Tracheal and Lung Surgery in Childhood, Obergurgl/Austria, January 1985

Harrison MR, Heldt GP, Brasch RC, de Lorimier AA, Gregory GA (1980) Resection of distal tracheal stenosis in a baby with agenesis of the lung. J Pediatr Surg 15:938

Heberer G, Schildberg FW, Valesky A, Stelter WJ (1980) Trachea-Rekonstruktionen bei entzündlichen Stenosen und Tumoren. Chirurg 51:283

Louhimo I, Leijala M (1985) Die Behandlung der präcarinalen Trachealstenose bei Neugeborenen und Kleinkindern. Paper presented at the 14th International Symposium: Tracheal and Lung Surgery in Childhood, Obergurgl/Austria, January 1985

Maeda M, Grillo HC (1973) Effect of tension on tracheal growth after resection and anastomosis in puppies. J Thorac Cardiovasc Surg 65:658

Mansfield PB (1980) Tracheal resection in infancy. J Pediatr Surg 15:79

Nakayama DK, Harrison MR, de Lorimier AA, Brasch RC, Fishman NH (1982) Reconstructive surgery for obstructing lesions of the intrathoracic trachea in infants and small children. J Pediatr Surg 17:854

O'Neill JA (1984) Experience with iatrogenic laryngeal and tracheal stenoses. J Pediatr Surg 19:
235
Salzer GM, Hartl H, Wurnig P (1985) Resektionsbehandlung bei Trachealstenosen im frühen
Kindesalter. Paper presented at the 14th International Symposium: Tracheal and Lung
Surgery in Childhood, Obergurgl/Austria, January 1985
Schildberg FW, Valesky A, Stelter WJ (1980a) Trachearesektionen und bronchoplastische Ein-
griffe bei Narbenstenosen, benignen und malignen Tumoren. Langenbecks Arch Chir 352:
281
Schildberg FW, Valesky A, Stelter WJ (1980b) Behandlung tumorbedingter und narbiger Tra-
chealstenosen. Münch Med Wochenschr 122:865

Treatment of Tracheal Stenoses
by Resection in Infancy and Early Childhood

G. M. Salzer[1], H. Hartl[2], and P. Wurnig[3]

Introduction

There are extraordinarily few publications on resection of tracheal stenoses in infancy and early childhood in the international literature. Various questions, such as resection versus longitudinal incision of the stenosis, the use of cardiopulmonary bypass e.t.c. are still the subjects of controversy, so that this sort of tracheal surgery must still be considered to be in an experimental stage. If a surgeon is confronted with one of these very rare cases, decisions must frequently be made on matters in which either very little experience is available or the literature contains no reports at all.

With regard to the planning of therapy it is not important whether the tracheal stenosis is congenital or a complication following long-term intubation or tracheostomy. It is not always easy to differentiate between these two forms if clear histological criteria are lacking, since congenital stenoses usually require emergency intubation and long-term ventilation before the cause of dyspnoea can be clarified.

There is general agreement that short tracheal stenoses should be treated by circumferential tracheal resection (Frisch et al. 1984; Harrison et al. 1980; Mansfield 1980; Nakayama et al. 1982; Wurnig and Hopfgartner 1978), but it has not been specified, in contrast to the situation in adults, what proportion of the trachea can be resected and still allow tension-free end-to-end anastomosis. In some cases the resection of 50% of the trachea has been possible (Debrand et al. 1979, Mattingly et al. 1981). In contrast, Idriss et al. (1984) recently performed anterior longitudinal incision of tracheal stenoses with plastic enlargement by free transplantation of a pericardial flap with cardiopulmonary bypass in five cases where at least a resection would have been possible. Their method has yielded good results with a follow-up period of 22 months so far.

Hypoplasias of the whole trachea were treated in one case by anterior (Kimura et al. 1982) and in another by posterior (Ein et al. 1982) plastic enlargement.

So far, circumferential tracheal resection has been performed in six infants and small children in Austria, as indicated by survey conducted among Austrian paediatric and thoracic surgeons.

[1]Department of Thoracic Surgery, Second University Hospital of Surgery, A-6020 Innsbruck, Austria.
[2]State Children's Hospital, A-4020 Linz, Austria.
[3]Mautner Markhof Children's Hospital of Vienna, A-1030 Vienna, Austria.

Progress in Pediatric Surgery, Vol. 21
Ed. by P. Wurnig
© Springer-Verlag Berlin Heidelberg 1987

Case Histories

Acquired Tracheal Stenoses

Case 1

Girl, 4 years; iatrogenic tracheal injury sustained during tracheostomy for false croup in another hospital with subsequent stenosis in the region of the tracheostomy. Resection (Wurnig) via collar incision 2 months later. Complication: granulations at the anastomotic ring, requiring excision. Extent of resection 30 mm. Final result: cure.

Case 2

Boy, 3.5 years; respiratory distress syndrome owing to prematurity (2100 g) necessitated intubation for 4 weeks. Development of a subglottic tracheal stenosis necessitating tracheostomy. Three years later resection of the stenosis (Hartl) via collar approach; end-to-end anastomosis while tracheal cannula still in place. Extent of resection 12 mm. Decannulation 4 weeks postoperatively. Final result: cure.

Case 3

Girl, 5 years; Long-term ventilation for false croup at the age of 1 year; subsequent development of a subglottic tracheal stenosis requiring tracheostomy. Four years later resection (Hartl) with the same technique as used in case 2. Final result: cure.

Congenital Tracheal Stenoses

Case 4

Boy, 4 months, velum-like tracheal malformation with cartilaginous defect immediately above the carina. Resection of the malformation (Wurnig) via right-sided transthoracic approach and end-to-end anastomosis. Length resected 14 mm. Ventilation during anastomosis via tracheal tube advanced into the right main bronchus. Complication: 6 weeks postoperatively asphyxia again, caused by complete expiratory collapse of the anastomotic region. Definitive stabilization of the trachea following ventilation for 3 weeks. Final result: cure. (This case has already been published by Wurnig and Hopfgartner [1978].)

Case 5

Girl, premature (1630 g); postpartal respiratory distress syndrome necessitated immediate intubation and ventilation; tracheography 4 months later revealed a circular stenosis in the midregion of the thoracic trachea. Resection (Salzer) via right transthoracic approach; length resected 13 mm. Intraoperative ventilation via tracheal tube advanced into the left main bronchus (Barclay et al. 1957), end-to-end anastomosis. Pathohistological examination led to the diagnosis of a congenital stenosis (hypertrophic bronchial glands in the submucosa and lining by multiply stratified squamous epithelium). Final result: cure. (This case has already been published by Frisch et al. [1984].)

Case 6

Girl, 4 months; congenital stenosis of the distal trachea extending from the jugulum downwards over the carina into the first 5 mm of both main bronchi. Resection (Salzer) of the entire stenosis including the carina; length resected 25 mm. Intraoperative ventilation via tracheal tube advanced into the left main bronchus. Reconstruction of the carina by junction of main bronchi by sutures, subsequent end-to-end anastomosis with the proximal trachea. Uneventful postoperative healing of the anastomosis. Repeated bronchoscopies did not show granulations in the anastomotic region. Complication: dyspnoea resulting in occasional airways infections required repeated intubation. This could possibly be due to paralysis of the recurrent nerve caused during surgery. After a fairly long period of normal respiration transfer to the district hospital 14 weeks postoperatively. A further episode of dyspnoea led to admission to another university E.N.T. clinic, where tracheostomy for paralysis of the recurrent nerve and bougienage of the anastomotic region because of granulations were performed. Artificial ventilation was continued. The child died 5 months postoperatively from a ventilator incident. There was no post-mortem examination and consequently no analysis of the state in the anastomotic region.

Five of the small children in whom circumferential tracheal resection was performed show that this kind of treatment can be applied with good results for both congenital and acquired tracheal stenoses. The fatal outcome in the sixth case, which was by far the most complicated, leaves the question of what therapy is best for extensive tracheal stenoses affecting both main bronchi open. Resection of the carina, which is technically feasible even in small children, cannot be recommended until there is more experience with these extremely rare cases.

Summary

An inquiry of Austrian paediatric and thoracic surgeons revealed six children aged 4 months to 5 years who had undergone circumferential resection of the trachea for congenital or acquired tracheal stenoses. Clinical data relating to these six Austrian cases are briefly presented. Experience shows that circumferential resection of localized tracheal stenoses can also be recommended for infants and young children.

Résumé

Une étude faite par des spécialistes autrichiens de la chirurgie infantile et de la chirurgie du thorax concerne 6 enfants âgés de 4 mois à 6 ans, ayant subi une résection transversale de la trachée pour remédier à une sténose congénitale ou acquise. Les données cliniques des six cas observés en Autriche sont brièvement présentées. L'expérience acquise a prouvé que la résection transversale dans le cas de sténose trachéales localisées peut très bien être pratiquée chez les petits enfants et les nourrissons.

Zusammenfassung

Aufgrund einer Umfrage unter den österreichischen Kinder- und Thoraxchirurgen wurden 6 Patienten im Alter von 4 Monaten bis 5 Jahren erfaßt, bei denen wegen angeborener oder erworbener Trachealstenosen eine Querresektion der Luftröhre durchgeführt wurde. Die klinischen Daten der 6 österreichischen Fälle werden kurz dargestellt. Die gewonnenen Erfahrungen zeigen, daß das Konzept der Kontinuitätsresektion umschriebener Trachealstenosen auch für das Säuglings- und Kleinkindalter empfohlen werden kann.

References

Barclay RS, McSwan M, Welsh TM (1957) Tracheal reconstruction without the use of grafts. Thorax 12:177–180
Debrand M, Tsueda, Browning SK, Wright BD, Todd EP (1979) Anesthesia for extensive resection of congenital tracheal stenosis in an infant. Anesth Analg 58:431–433
Ein SH, Friedberg J, Williams WG, Rearon B, Barker GA, Mancher K (1982) Tracheoplasty – a new operation for complete congenital tracheal stenosis. J Pediatr Surg 17:872–878
Frisch H, Salzer GM, Berger H, Luz O, Pastner E, Fink M, Kroesen G, Spoendlin H, Mikuz G (1984) Die Trachealstenose nach Langzeitintubation des Neugeborenen und ihre operative Korrektur. Paediatr Prax 30:379–385
Harrison MR, Heldt GP, Brasch RC, Lorimier AA, Gregory GA (1980) Resection of distal tracheal stenosis in a baby with agenesis of the lung. J Pediatr Surg 15:938–943
Idriss FS, Deleon SY, Ilbawi MN, Gerson CR, Tucker GF, Holinger F (1984) Tracheoplasty with pericardial patch for extensive tracheal stenosis in infants and children. J Thorac Cardiovasc Surg 88:527–536
Kimura K, Mukohara N, Tsugawa C, Matsumoto Y, Sugimura C, Murata H, Itoh H (1982) Tracheoplasty for congenital stenosis of the entire trachea. J Pediatr Surg 17:869–871
Mansfield PB (1980) Tracheal resection in infancy. J Pediatr Surg 15:79–81
Mattingly WT, Belin RP, Todd EP (1981) Surgical repair of congenital tracheal stenosis in an infant. J Thorac Cardiovasc Surg 81:738–740
Nakayama DK, Harrison MR, Lorimier AA, Brasch RC, Fishman NH (1982) Reconstructive surgery for obsructing lesions of the intrathoracic trachea in infants and small children. J Pediatr Surg 17:854–868
Wurnig P, Hopfgartner L (1978) Korrelation bronchoskopischer und röntgenologischer Befunde im Kindesalter. Pädiatr Fortbild K Praxis 46:48–63

Long-Distance Resection of the Trachea with Primary Anastomosis in Small Children

H. Halsband[1]

It was as long ago as 1896 when von Eiselsberg averred that it was possible to re-sect tracheal stenoses.

In 1958, Dor and Carcassonne published an experimental study on tracheo-plasties in 120 dogs, in which they, too, described tracheal resection with primary anastomosis as the most suitable method of treating tracheal stenoses.

Nevertheless, during the early 1960s reconstructive plastic methods were pre-ferred for the treatment of congenital and acquired stenoses of the upper respira-tory tract.

It was not until the mid-1960s that segmental resection of the trachea for the correction of acquired tracheal stenoses in *adults* found increasing acceptance as the treatment of choice; Grillo's group (Grillo et al. 1964; Mulliken and Grillo 1968) and Naef (1972) have shown that it is possible to resect more than 50% of the tracheal length and carry out a primary anastomosis of the tracheal stumps in adults; in practical terms, 30% of the tracheal length can be resected if the normal position of the head is maintained after the operation, and a further 17% if exten-sive mobilization of the tracheal stumps is accomplished during the operation and the head is positioned at 30° flexion postoperatively.

Additional mobilization of the neighbouring organs, such as larynx, lungs and vessels, has made it possible in individual cases to perform resections of up to a total length of 7–8 cm, which is a total of seven to nine tracheal rings. This tracheal gap corresponds to approx. 70% of the total tracheal length in adults.

Experience in tracheal resection in adults has meanwhile been documented in an extensive literature: in all 661 tracheal resections were described in the interna-tional literature by 52 authors from 1896 to 1980 (Valesky 1980); 585 of these in-volved the proximal trachea and 76, the distal trachea and the bifurcation.

In contrast, only 26 case reports dealing with segmental resection of the trachea in *children* (up to the age of 16) were found in the literature, all published between 1969 and 1984 (Jewsbury 1969; Louhimo et al. 1971; Carcassonne et al. 1973; Sørensen 1974; Kornmesser 1974; Pearson et al. 1974; Schoefer 1975; Grillo 1979; Mansfield, cited in Grillo 1979; Moritz and Schlick 1979; Halsband and Valesky 1981; Frisch et al. 1984). The postoperative courses, however, are in-adequately documented or not at all, so that the publications available do not

---

[1]Paediatric Surgical Clinic, Medical University of Lübeck, Kahlhorststrasse 31–35, D-2400 Lübeck, FRG.

Progress in Pediatric Surgery, Vol. 21
Ed. by P. Wurnig
© Springer-Verlag Berlin Heidelberg 1987

Table 1. Complications of tracheal resection with primary anastomosis

---

1. Suture failure/leakage of the anastomosis
   → Permanent tracheostomy

2. Wound healing disturbances/infections
   → Rupture of the anastomosis
   → Permanent tracheostomy

3. Vascular erosion/haemorrhage

4. Paresis of recurrent laryngeal nerves

5. Disturbance of growth/granulation tissue at the suture line
   → Restenosis

6. Mortality in adults: 5% (−10%)

---

allow any general conclusions as to whether the procedure is truly appropriate in children.

More wide-spread application of segmental resection of the trachea in children has been prevented in the past by fears of

Suture failure as a result of the increased tension exerted on the anastomosis, which appears even after resection of short-distance tracheal resections
Interference with growth with the necessity for subsequent restenosis
Technical difficulties arising from the smaller tracheal lumen in children, since marked cicatricial bulges might cause further problems by forming secondary stenoses
Other complications (see Table 1)

With reference to the question of restenosis with growth, Maeda and Grillo (1972) showed in an experimental study on tracheal resection carried out in puppies that the cross section of the tracheal lumen was 80% of normal when they were full-grown.

The most frequent treatment for congenital and acquired stenoses in the upper respiratory tract in children (both laryngostenosis especially cricoid stenosis, and tracheal stenosis) used to be dilatation plasty. However, these reconstructive methods require several operations over a lengthy period and involve the problems connected with the treatment of an organ in the process of growing.

The *advantages of segmental tracheal resection* with primary anastomosis over these methods are:

Preservation of the normal wall structure
One-stage procedure
Applicability in cases of tracheal stenosis in the cervical region and within the thorax, which cannot be corrected by dilatation plasty

Increased anastomotic tension is present even after resection of short circular tracheal segments and does not necessarily have a negative influence on wound healing with suture failure or stenosis. Animal experiments have shown, surprisingly (Valesky 1980), that it can even lead to a significantly stronger scar and problem-free healing: After resection of approx. 30% of the trachea in dogs the tensile strength of the anastomosis was approx. 170% of that of a normal tracheal tissue 8 weeks after surgery, and was thus three times higher than the tensile strength after simple severance without resection with no increased initial anastomotic tension. Polyglycol acid has proved to be the best suture material.

Operative Technique

The following aspects have to be taken into account when tracheal resection with primary anastomosis is carried out (Fig. 1):

– Oxygenation during resection of the stenosis and performance of the posterior suture of the anastomosis is ensured by means of a tube inserted directly from the operating field into the caudal tracheal stump. Before anastomosis of the anterior wall this tube is replaced by the nasopharyngeal tube, which is pushed down again.

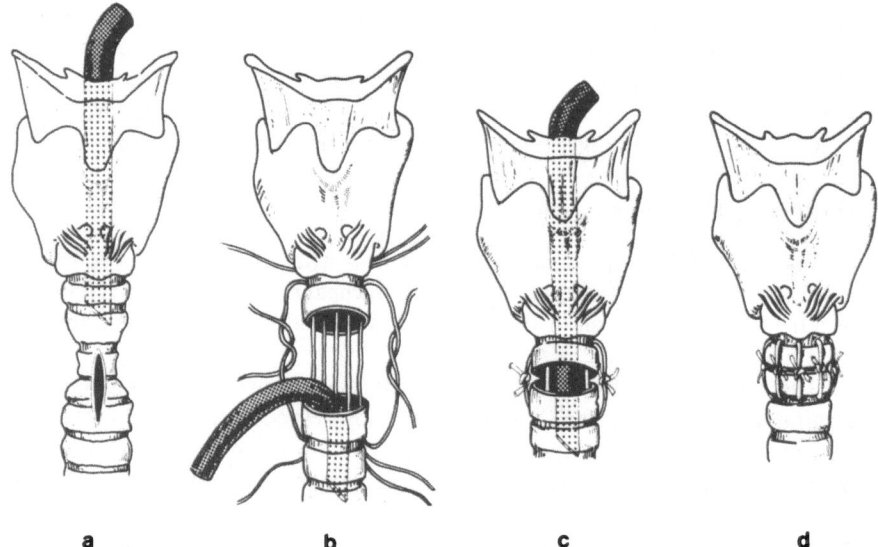

    a   **b**   **c**   **d**

Fig. 1a–d. Technique of tracheal resection with primary anastomosis. **a** Intubation by passage of tube through stenosis or insertion of tube above stenosis; extensive dissection of the trachea ventrally and dorsally, but only limited laterally. **b** After tracheal dissection direct intubation into the caudal tracheal stump across the operating field. Resection of the stenotic and fibrotic segment of the trachea and anastomosis of the posterior circumference with pericartilaginous transmucous stitches (absorbable ooo or oooo thread). **c** On completion of suture of posterior wall, insertion of nasopharyngeal tube into caudal stump of trachea. **d** Completion of the anastomosis

- Mobilization of the trachea should be limited to the anterior and posterior tracheal walls. Circular dissection involves the risk of an inadequate blood supply with subsequent wall necrosis, as the blood supply to the trachea is ensured by a lateral longitudinal vascular anastomosis whose intercartilaginous arterial branches supply the submucous capillary plexus with blood (Salassa et al. 1977; Muira and Grillo 1966).
- The strictured and fibrous region must be completely resected. Only cartilages with normal blood supply are suitable for anastomosis.
- To avoid paralysis of recurrent laryngeal nerves, preparation of a cicatricial stenosis should be carried out very close to the trachea, and a preparation of the vocal nerves in the mostly cicatricial part of the tissue should not be made at all.
- In our experience, the anastomosis is best sutured with pericartilaginous and transmucous stitches in absorbable suture material. These stitches avoid cuts by the sutures even when the tensile stress exerted on the anastomosis is extreme.
- Prolonged nasotracheal intubation is needed for some days postoperatively, as is positioning of the head at 30° flexion to reduce anastomotic tension.

Case Reports

Following the technique described above we have carried out long-distance tracheal resections involving four or five cartilaginous rings in three children aged 2½ to 4¾ years (Table 2).

This first case has already been reported (Halsband and Valesky 1981).

All three children were born prematurely and suffered from respiratory distress. After prolonged intubation for 5–9 months, the infants developed proximal tracheal stenoses, which necessitated tracheostomy in each. Repeated attempts at decannulation failed.

Case 1

This girl had a birth weight of 2200 g, and after 6 months' intubation and subsequent tracheostomy she developed an additional stomastenosis. The total length of the stenotic tracheal section was 2.5 cm (Fig. 2a).

After complete healing of the inflammatory changes in the trachea, resection of the stenosis was performed when the girl was 2¾ years old. A total of five tracheal rings were resected and primary anastomosis was carried out. Postoperative intubation and ventilation were maintained for 1 week with the head in a flexed position. The course of healing was uneventful.

Several follow-up examinations revealed no clinical, radiological or endoscopical signs of restenosis (Fig. 2b).

The endoscopic studies confirmed that the anastomosis could only be recognized by a slight irregularity of the scar; there was no narrowing of the lumen and

Table 2. Long tracheal resections (personal experience)

Patient no. (sex)	History		Diagnosis	Resection		Course
	Birth weight	Intubation time (months) before tracheotomy		Age	Length	
1 (girl)	2200	6	Proximal tracheal stenosis + stoma malacia	2¾ years	5 tracheal rings (2–6)	Result excellent at 5 years after surgery
2 (girl)	1320	5	Subglottic stenosis	4¾ years	4 tracheal rings (2–5)	Result excellent at 2 years after surgery
3 (boy)	1670	9	Cricoid and proximal tracheal stenosis	2½ years	Ventral half of cricoid + 4 tracheal rings (1–4)	Normal at 2 months after surgery then cricoid restenosis requiring second tracheostomy

no instability of the wall, at the anastomotic site. The operation took place 5 years ago and the girl is now almost 8 years of age. She has made up for a deficit in her speech development and has no problems whatsoever with her upper respiratory tract. The development thus far encourages us to hope that no difficulties will arise in the course of further growth.

Case 2

This premature infant was a twin, with a birth weight of 1320 g. Long-term intubation and continuous ventilation over 5 months were necessary before she was tracheostomized. She was subject to severe bronchopulmonary dysplasia and recurrent bronchopneumonias.

Laryngotracheoscopy (Fig. 3a) at the age of 4¾ years revealed subglottic tracheomalacia over a length of 2½ cm, extending to the stoma. Decannulation was not possible. Therefore, the tracheal stenosis was resected with the region of the tracheostomy and the two proximal cartilaginous rings, making four rings in all. The postoperative follow-up tracheoscopies (Fig. 3b) revealed that the anastomosis had a cross section corresponding to the lumen in the rest of the tracheal. The anastomotic site proved to be as stable as the distal tracheal region. Clinically and radiologically no signs of restenosis were discovered in this child 2 years after the operation at the age of 7, and the result is very good.

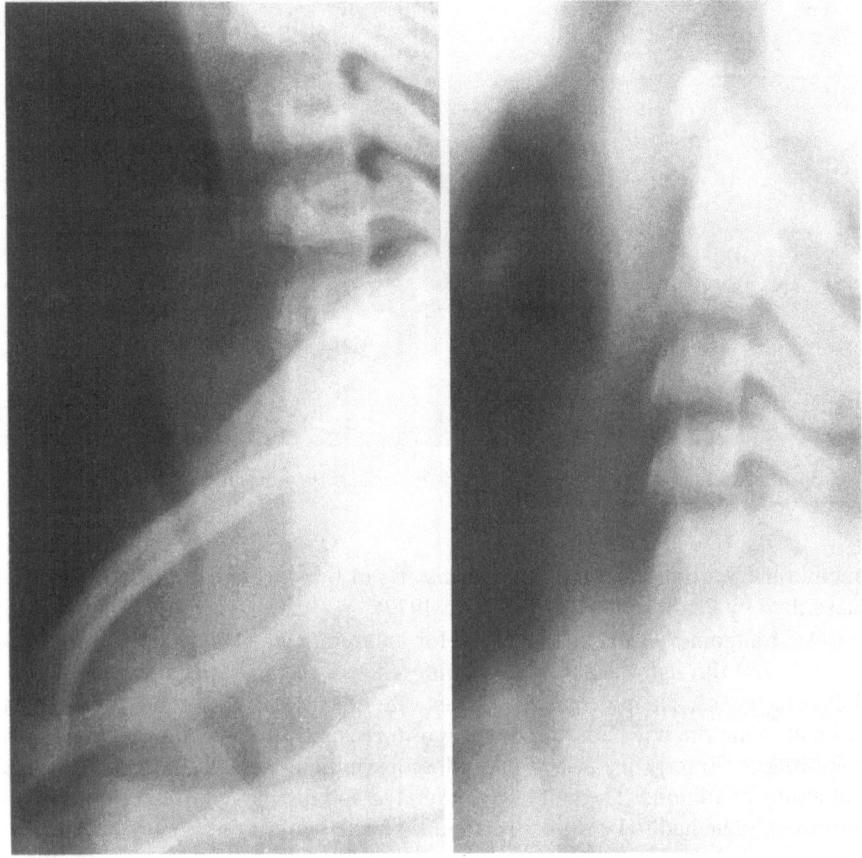

Fig. 2a, b. Case 1: **a** Preoperative radiogram of the tracheal stenosis approx. 2.5 cm in length; **b** 1 year after resection and primary anastomosis

Case 3

This premature male infant weighed 1670 g at birth. After 9 months' intubation and tracheostomy he had to wear a silver tracheal cannula until he underwent resection of a stenosis at the age of 2½ years. The preoperative endoscopic examination showed a conical high-grade stenosis below the vocal cords. The larynx could only be passed with the aid of the 3.0 tracheobronchoscopy shaft (Storz). The operation revealed extremely compact cicatrization of the proximal tracheal wall and the stoma region, as well as an hour glass-shaped stricture at the level of the first tracheal ring extending to the cricoid cartilage.

The proximal tracheal portion with four rings was resected together with the ventral circumference of the fibrous and undilatable cricoid cartilage; a primary anastomosis was carried out between the fifth tracheal ring and the cricothyroid

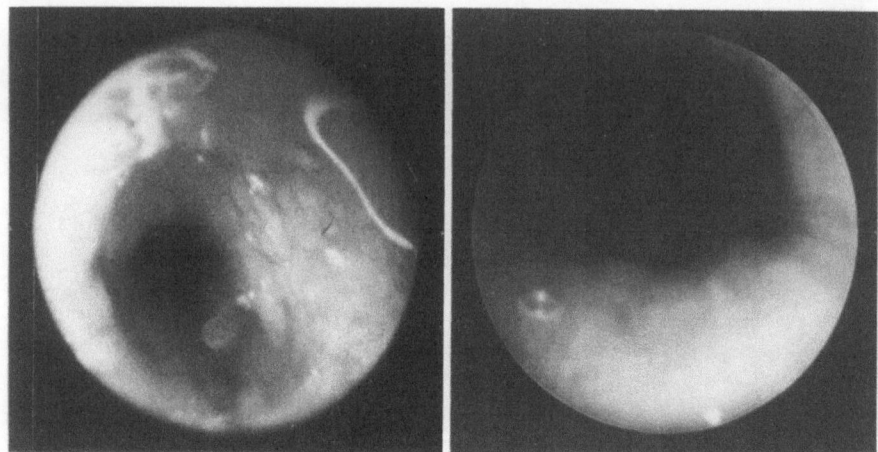

a   b

Fig. 3a, b. Case 2: **a** Subglottic tracheal stenosis/malacia; **b** 1¼ years after tracheal resection and
anastomosis

membrane ventrally and the remaining parts of the cricoid cartilage dorsally (as
described by Pearson et al. 1975; Grillo 1979).

A Montgomery tube was inserted for splinting. The T arm of the tube was
brought out through the anterior circumference of the anastomosis, where it was
left for 3 weeks. The postoperative phase was uneventful. However, after a short
time at home the boy had a sudden respiratory standstill following a quarrel with
his brother. Emergency follow-up endoscopy initially revealed sufficiently wide
subglottic conditions. The child was extubated and discharged from hospital. Un-
fortunately, he had to be retracheostomized because of further dyspnoeic attacks.
A restenosis had developed in the cricoid region. Perhaps the Montgomery tube,
which had been brought out in this anterior part of the anastomosis and caused a
certain defect, was responsible for development of the second stenosis.

While the tracheal stenosis in this child was also corrected by a resection, the
procedure was inadequate for the cricoid stenosis. The combination of tracheal
resection and anastomosis with a cricoid dilatation procedure according to the
Zürich method (Hof et al.) would have avoided the new cricoid stenosis.

Conclusions

Our experience with long tracheal resections in children is limited to three cases
in small children of 2½ to 4¾ years. The results described above encourage us to
recommend the treatment of isolated tracheal stenoses by continuity resection
also in children. This procedure ensures successful lasting removal of even long
stenoses. The chief requirements are correct indication and technique. If an additional laryngostenosis is found, combination with cricoid resection or cricoid cartilage dilatation is recommended.

Summary

While tracheal resection with primary anastomosis has been accepted as the therapy of choice for tracheal stenoses in adults since the 1960s, only 26 case reports are available on continuity resections of the trachea in children. The advantages of continuity resection include the one-stage procedure and the preservation of the natural wall structures. Anastomosis should be accomplished with pericartilaginous sutures and absorbable suture material. The increased tension on anastomoses inserted following resection of long tracheal segments does not necessarily have a negative influence on wound healing. The case histories of three small children are given in this report: they all underwent tracheal continuity resections involving four or five rings because of postintubation stenoses. The results of resection after up to 5 years' follow-up are very good, so that this method can be recommended in preference to the reconstructive tracheoplasty in children, which takes longer.

If the cricoid cartilage is also involved a combination of tracheal resection and cricoid resection/dilatation is recommended.

Résumé

Alors que la résection trachéale avec anastomose primaire a fait ses preuves et est la méthode de choix pour le traitement des sténoses trachéales des adultes depuis les années 60, il n'existe que 26 observations de cas de résections trachéales en continuité chez des enfants. Avantages de la résection en continuité: procédure en un temps et préservation des structures naturelles des parois. L'anastomose doit être faite avec des sutures péricartilagineuses et un fil résorbable. L'augmentation de la tension de l'anastomose lors d'une longue résection n'est pas obligatoirement péjorative pour la guérison de la plaie. On a observé 3 cas de petits enfants ayant subi une résection en continuité de 4 ou 5 anneaux pour traitement de sténoses après intubation. Les résultats (patients suivis jusqu'à 5 ans après l'intervention) sont très bons et permettent d'affirmer que cette méthode est préférable à la reconstruction plastique de la trachée chez les enfants.

Si le cartilage cricoïde est atteint, il est recommandé de combiner une résection trachéale et une résection/dilatation du cricoïde.

Zusammenfassung

Während sich bei Erwachsenen seit den 60er Jahren zur Behandlung von Trachealstenosen die Resektion mit primärer Anastomose als die Therapie der Wahl bewährt hat, liegen über Kontinuitätsresektionen der Trachea bei Kindern bisher nur 26 Fallberichte vor.

Die Vorteile der Kontinuitätsresektion bestehen im einseitigen Vorgehen sowie in der Erhaltung der natürlichen Wandstrukturen. Die Anastomosennaht sollte nach der eigenen Erfahrung perikartilaginär unter Verwendung von resorbierbarem Nahtmaterial erfolgen. Die bei langstreckiger Resektion auftretende erhöhte Anastomosenspannung führt nicht zwangsläufig zu einer negativen Beeinflussung der Wundheilung.

Es wird über 3 Kleinkinder berichtet, bei denen wegen postintubationsbedingter Trachealstenosen Kontinuitätsresektionen von 4–5 Ringen durchgeführt wurden. Die Resektionsergebnisse – bis 5 Jahre postoperativ – sind sehr gut, so daß diese Methode gegenüber den längere Zeit dauernden rekonstruktiv-plastischen Verfahren bei Kindern vorzugsweise empfohlen werden kann.

Bei Mitbetroffenheit des Ringknorpels empfiehlt sich eine Kombination von Trachealresektion und krikoiderweiternden/resezierenden Verfahren.

References

Carcassonne M, Dor V, Aubert J, Kreitmann P (1973) Tracheal resection with primary anastomosis in children. J Pediatr Surg 8:1–8

Dor J, Carcassonne M (1958) Contribution expérimentale à la réparation des pertes de substance de la trachée et des bronches. Ann Chir 12:1041–1048

Eiselsberg A von (1896) Zur Resection und Naht der Trachea. Dtsch Med Wochenschr 22:343–344

Frisch H, Salzer G-M, Kroesen G, Berger H, Luz O (1984) Die Trachealstenose nach Langzeit-Intubation und ihre operative Korrektur. Paper presented at the Symposium on Paediatric Intensive Care, Berlin, April 1984

Grillo HC (1979) Surgical treatment of postintubation tracheal injuries. J Thorac Cardiovasc Surg 78:860–875

Grillo HC, Dignan EF, Miura T (1964) Extensive resection and reconstruction of mediastinal trachea without prosthesis or graft: an anatomical study in man. J Thorac Cardiovasc Surg 48:741–749

Halsband H, Valesky A (1981) Trachealresektion im Kindesalter. Paper presented at the Annual Congress of the Deutsche Gesellschaft für Kinderheilkunde and the Deutsche Gesellschaft für Kinderchirurgie, Düsseldorf, September 1981

Halsband H, Valesky A (1984) Trachea-Kontinuitäts-Resektion im frühen Kindesalter. Paper presented at the Symposium on Pediatric Intensive Care, Berlin, April 1984

Hof E, Grossenbacher R, Fisch U (1978) Ergebnisse der operativen Versorgung laryngotrachealer Stenosen. HNO 26:60–64

Jewsbury P (1969) Resection of tracheal stricture following tracheostomy. Lancet 2:411–413

Kornmesser HJ (1974) Segmentresektion der Trachea im Kindesalter. Laryng Rhinol 53:395–398

Louhimo J, Grahne B, Parila M, Suntarinen T (1971) Acquired laryngotracheal stenosis in children. J Pediatr Surg 6:730–737

Maeda M, Grillo HC (1972) Tracheal growth following anastomosis in puppies. J Thorac Cardiovasc Surg 64:304–313

Miura T, Grillo HC (1966) The contribution of the inferior thyroid pole to the blood supply of the human trachea. Surg Gynecol Obstet 123:99–102

Moritz E, Schlick W (1979) Spätergebnisse nach Trachealresektion. Wien Klin Wochenschr 91:97–101

Mulliken JB, Grillo HC (1968) The limits of tracheal resection with primary anastomosis: further anatomical studies in man. J Thorac Cardiovasc Surg 55:418–421

Naef AP (1972) Tracheobronchialresektion. Thoraxchir 20:283–285

Pearson FG, Thompson DW, Weissberg D, Simpson WJK, Kergin FG (1974) Adenoid cystic carcinoma of the trachea; experience with 16 patients managed by tracheal resection. Ann Thorac Surg 18:16–27

Pearson FG, Cooper JD, Nelems JM, Vannostrand AWP (1975) Primary tracheal anastomosis after resection of cricoid cartilage with preservation of recurrent laryngeal nerves. J Thorac Cardiovasc Surg 70:806–816

Salassa JR, Pearson FG, Payne WS (1977) Gross and microscopic blood supply of the trachea. Ann Thorac Surg 23:100–107

Schoefer G (1975) Resektionen der Trachea und Bifurkation. Zentralbl Chir 100:277–289

Sørensen HR (1974) Circular resection of the trachea for malignant and benign diseases. J Franc Otorhinolaryng 23:400–402

Valesky A (1980) Die Kontinuitätsresektion der Trachea; ein experimenteller und klinischer Beitrag zur Behandlung obstruierender Trachealerkrankungen. Thesis, Lübeck

Zenker R, Schaudig A, Pichlmaier H (1972) Gegenwärtiger Stand der Resektion von Trachea und Bronchien. MMW 114:1090

Clinical Symptoms and Therapy of Lung Separation

K. Gdanietz[1], K. Vorpahl[2], G. Piehl[1], and A. Höck[3]

Introduction

Lung separation is an anomaly of the lung characterized by three anatomical entities: abnormal arterial blood supply, bronchial anomaly and parenchymatous dysgenesis. Aetiologically, an embryonic maldevelopment is responsible. Numerous explanations have been suggested (Table 1). If the malformed part of the lung is located within a lung lobe or segment it is referred to as intralobar separation (Fig. 1), while the term extralobar separation is used if it is separated from the lung (Fig. 2). This lung anomaly has been described by different terms (Table 2). The most common is "sequestration", which was introduced into medical terminology by Pryce (1946) for the intralobar forms. This term, however, does not really mean a malformation, and it has therefore repeatedly been questioned in

Table 1. Explanations suggested for the aetiology of so-called lung separations and lung sequestrations

Year	Author and theory
1861	Rektorzik
	Fraction theory: separation of normally developed lung
1878	Ruge
	Excess theory: ingrowth of the foregut, development of a rudimentary 3rd lung
1946	Pryce
	Traction theory: separate artery runs to the embryonal lung-anlage
1950	Smith
	Blood supply theory: parenchymatous changes induced by insufficient arterial blood supply
1958	Boyden
	Coincidental occurrence theory: simultaneous appearance of arterial and parenchymatous malformation
1959	Gebauer and Mason
	Theory of acquired anomalies: result of recurrent infections

[1]Paediatric Surgical Clinic, [2]Second Pathological Institute, and [3]Second Paediatric Clinic of the Klinikum Berlin-Buch, DDR-1115 Berlin-Buch, GDR.

Progress in Pediatric Surgery, Vol. 21
Ed. by P. Wurnig
© Springer-Verlag Berlin Heidelberg 1987

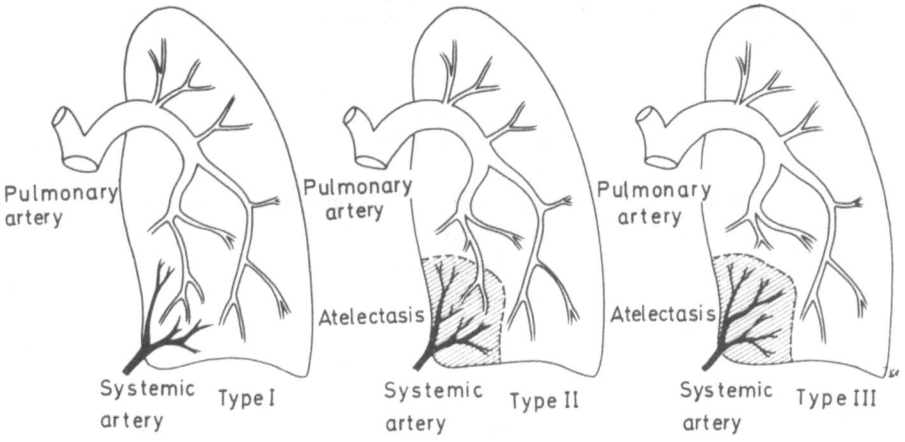

Fig. 1. Types of intralobar separation or sequestration according to Pryce (1946). (From Bettex et al. 1981)

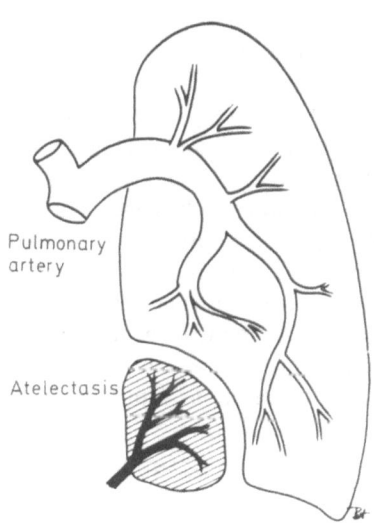

Fig. 2. Extralobar separation or sequestration according to Gray and Skandalakis (1972). (From Bettex et al. 1981)

the german literature. It defines dead, formerly functioning and demarcated tissue. Whereas other authors generally describe variants of form and location (Hasche 1962; Herxheimer 1901; Huber 1777; Kaup 1891; Rektorzik 1861; Rokitansky 1861; Ruge 1878; Springer 1898), Engelmann (1976) relates the term "lung malformation with abnormal haemodynamics" to the nosological unit of bronchopulmonary and pulmonary vascular malformation. He recommends this term, with the argument that "the mutual factor is not really the organic malformation of the latter, but rather the always observably abnormal connection of the

Table 2. Names given to lung anomalies with bronchopulmonary and pulmonary vascular malformations

Year	Author	Name
1777	Huber	Accessory lung lobe
1861	Rokitansky	Lobe
1891	Kaup	Diaphragmatic hernia with separation of a lung part
1898	Springer	Rudimentary accessory lung
1901	Herxheimer	True accessory lung
1903	Voisin	Aberrant lobe
1962	Hasche	Separation
1972	Stöcker	Separation
1946	Pryce	Sequestration
1976	Engelmann	Lung malformation with abnormal haemodynamics

lung or part of it with the systemic circulation or a bypass between systemic and pulmonary circulation".

Whereas the blood flow normally follows a right-left shunt, it represents a left-left shunt in intralobar separation and a left-right shunt in extralobar separation (Engelmann 1976), Both forms have their own blood supply. The systemic arteries originate either from the thoracic aorta or from the abdominal aorta above the coeliac trunk, or the intercoastal arteries. Venous return ensues via the azygos and left azygos or the portal vein. Histologically, aeration can be concluded from expanded alveoli and bronchi. Congenital connection with a bronchus is assumed in 20% of cases of the intralobar form. Air entry via inflammatory changes is another explanation put forward. Actually, there should be no connections with the respiratory tract in extralobar forms. Nevertheless, connections with trachea and bronchi were described in 1972 by Gray and Skandalakis and in 1975 by Halil and Kilman, and we are able to add a third case. Connections with oesophagus and stomach exist in both intra- and extralobar forms.

Localization

Intralobar separations are most commonly located in the posterolateral segments of the left lower lung lobe, and extralobar forms also most often affect the left lower lobe. Infra- and subdiaphragmatic localization and involvement of the apical segment of the upper lung lobe, involvement of the whole lung and bilateral intralobar separations have been described (Voisin 1903). In 1983 Schwartz et al. published a case of total lung sequestration associated with oesophageal atresia and multiple oesophagotracheal fistulas. The infant survived when it had undergone gastrostomy, left-sided thoracotomy with division of oesophagotracheal fistulas and oesophageal anastomosis and right-sided pneumonectomy.

Clinical Symptoms

Lung separations have also been described in advanced old age. They become clinically manifest if complications occur. The most frequent complications are infections, such as recurrent bronchopneumonia or recurrent infection of the same segment, particularly the posterobasal segment of the left lower lung lobe affected by a lung separation detected at differential diagnosis. Changed haemodynamics in cardiac malformations leading to excessive blood supply and subsequent cardiac decompensation are rarely seen in lung separations.

Diagnosis

Diagnosis is made by clinical and radiological examination. Retro- and paracardiac infiltrations are seen in the lower lung lobe, which sometimes contains cystic structures. Chest X-ray does not allow differentiation between intra- and extralobar separation and cysts of other origins. Connections with the gastrointestinal tract are excluded by an upper GI X-ray series. Bronchography allows classification into types I, II and III according to Pryce (1946) for intralobar forms (Fig. 1) and according to Gray and Skandalakis (1972) for extralobar forms (Fig. 2). Angiography reveals the origin of the systemic arteries supplying the lung separation, and not until this has been done the diagnosis can be regarded as definitive.

Indications for Operation

Indications for operation result from possible infections and the complications of possible cardiac insufficiency. Genton (1981) recommends immediate operation once the diagnosis is established.

Therapy

The treatment of choice is surgery, based on the following considerations:

1. Resection of the separated part of the lung if diagnosis was made incidentally, which is sometimes the case in diaphragmatic relaxation.
2. Resection of the separated part of the lung if there is associated congenital heart disease. Both malformations can be corrected in a single session.
3. Resection of the separated part of the lung if there are clinical symptoms with recurrent infections of the same localization, particularly of the lower lobe.

Operative Technique

First the arteries are looked for and ligated, then the veins, followed by segmental or lobar resection. Removal of extralobar separations is usually easy.

The risk involved in the operation is low if it is performed by a surgeon experienced in thoracic surgery. The postoperative course is usually uneventful.

Personal Cases

From 1960 to 1985 we operated on nine patients with lung separation (Table 3). The clinical symptoms were stridor in one case and pulmonary complaints in three (suspected tumour in two): in four cases the lung separation was an incidental

Table 3. Authors' own cases of lung separation (1963–1985)

Case no.	Sex	Year of operation	Age at time of operation	Type: ELS/ILS	Localization	Diagnosis
1	Girl	1963	16 days	ILS	Left epi-diaphragmatic	Incidental finding in diaphragmatic relaxation
2	Girl	1965	8 months	ELS	Left epi-diaphragmatic	Incidental finding in diaphragmatic relaxation
3	Boy	1970	24 days	ELS	Left epi-diaphragmatic	Incidental finding in diaphragmatic relaxation
4	Boy	1970	9 days	ELS	Right upper lobe	Tumour suspected
5	Boy	1975	9 months	ILS	Left lower lobe	Preoperatively diagnosed
6	Girl	1975	2 years, 10 months	ELS	Right upper lobe	Tumour suspected
7	Girl	1979	1 day	ELS	Left epi-diaphragmatic	Incidental finding in ruptured diaphragmatic hernia on the left-hand side
8	Girl	1966	2 days	ILS	Left lower lobe	Incidental finding in diaphragmatic relaxation
9	Girl	1985	4 months	ELS	Right pleural cavity	Recurrent right-sided pleural effusion; tumour suspected

ELS, extralobar separation; ILS, intralobar separation

finding in a left-sided diaphragmatic relaxation; and recurrent pleural effusions leading to suspicion of a tumour were observed in one. Separations were interlobar in three cases, all in the left lower lobe. In six they were extralobar, three of them by the left lower lobe, two by the right upper lobe, and one by the middle lobe. There was no connection with the gastrointestinal tract in any case. Preoperative angiography was carried out in only one case, since thoracotomy was performed for suspected tumours in three cases and separations were incidental findings in six. In case 9 (Table 3) an extralobar separation was found which had a connection with the tracheobronchial system. In this child a right-sided hydrothorax was diagnosed prenatally by ultrasound and confirmed postnatally by chest X-ray (Fig. 3). Repeated pleural effusions were yellowish and clear, odourless and sterile. Further radiological examination (Fig. 4), CT scans and ultrasound tomography revealed a solid area 4.5 cm in diameter above the right diaphragm, paracardially and paravertebrally situated within the pleural effusion.

A more detailed presentation of this case from the obstetric and neonatological viewpoint will be published separately.

Thoracotomy was performed on 12 March 1985, under the tentative diagnosis intrathoracic tumour of unknown origin. After aspiration of the pleural effusion a

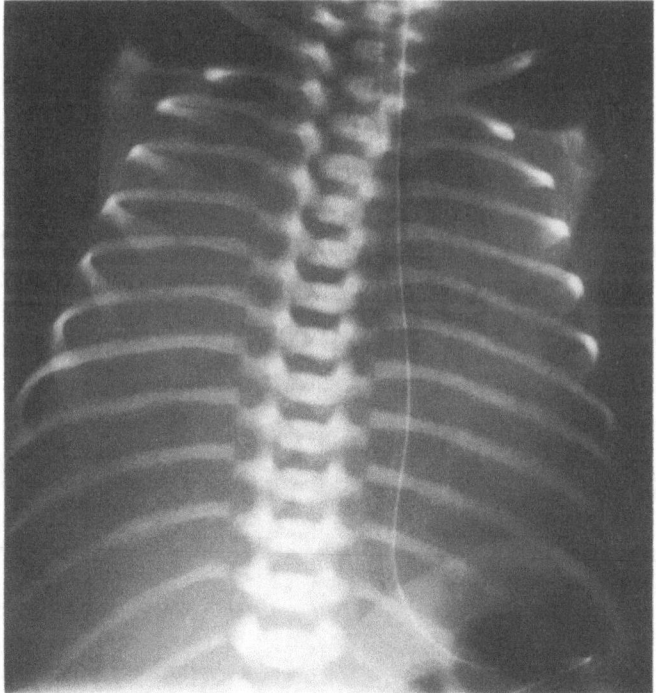

Fig. 3. Chest X-ray on the day of birth (9 Nov. 1984). Opacity in the whole of the right hemithorax (case 9)

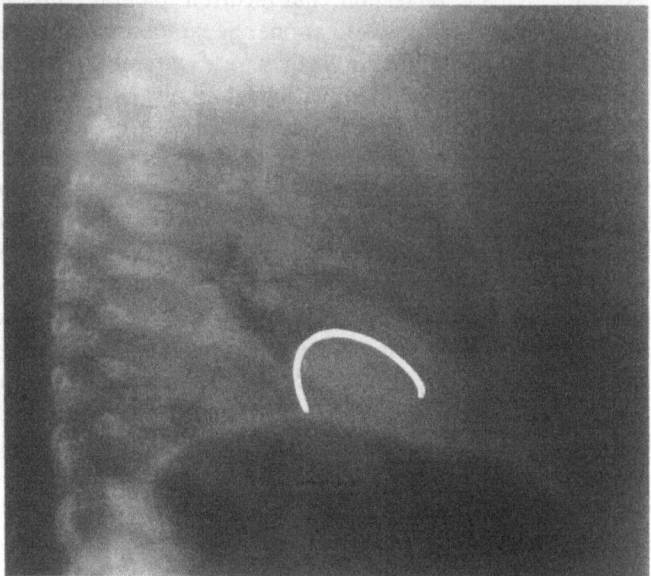

Fig. 4. Chest X-ray in lateral view 7 days before thoracotomy. Only weak opacity above the right diaphragm (contours marked)

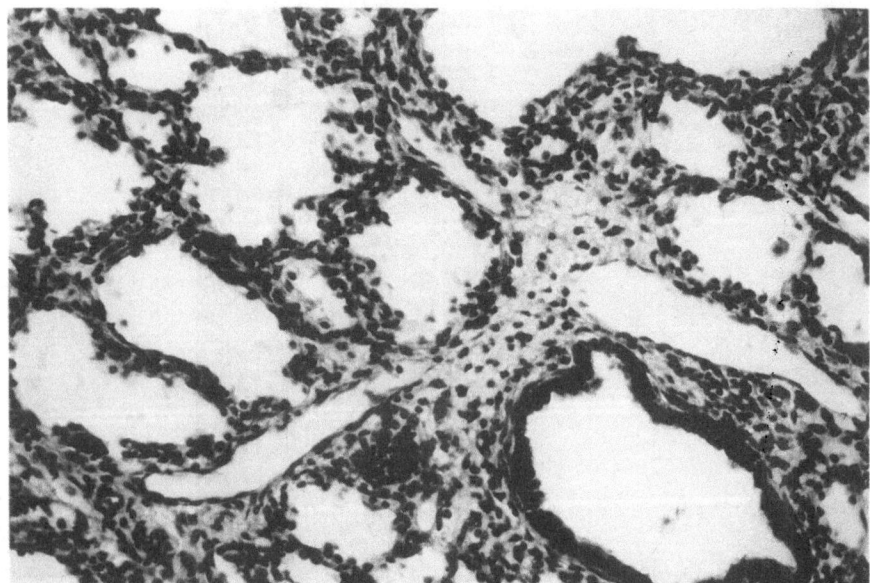

Fig. 5. Almost complete alveolar unfolding. A bronchiolus is seen at the lower rim of the picture. H & E, × 320

$4 \times 4 \times 2$ cm sized, smooth, round, pediculated, pink tumour was found, which was covered by pleura. The lobar structure of the lung was normal. The tumour pedicle was pencil-shaped and was inserted to the right of the vertebral column at the level of the 9th vertebral body and contained blood vessels. The pedicle was sutured, ligated and transected.

Pathohistological Findings

Lung tissue with partly unfolded alveoli was found, the alveolar lumina optically empty but containing isolated shed alveolar cover cells (Fig. 5); there was no evidence of aspiration of foreign material, and atelectases and inflammatory changes were also absent; the alveolar walls slightly enlarged; numerous, partly ectatic bronchi and bronchioli with regular wall structure were present; pleura was markedly enlarged and fibrosed; below the mesothelium there were numerous, considerably ectatic lymph vessels (Fig. 6) and ectatic peribronchial lymph vessels.

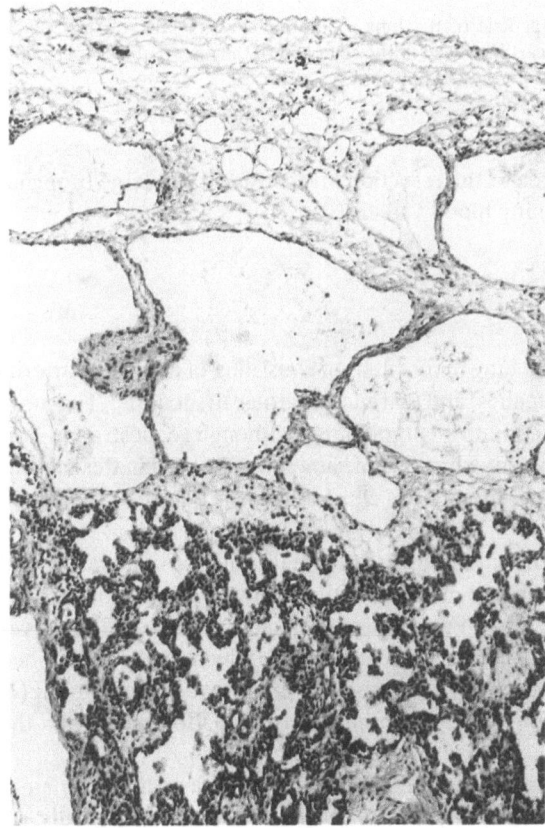

Fig. 6. Considerably enlarged pleura and ectatic lymph vessels seen in the upper half of the picture. Inadequately ventilated lung parenchyma below. H&E, × 125

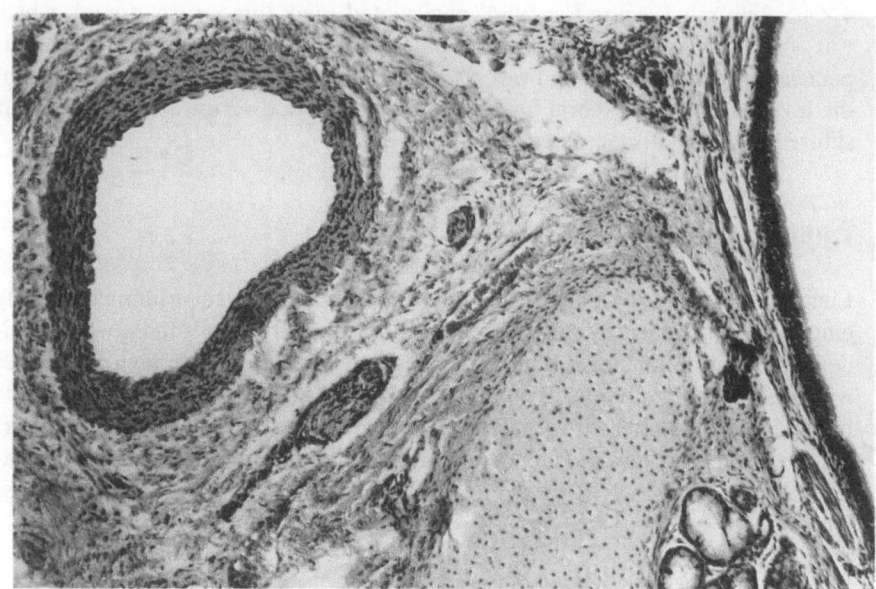

Fig. 7. Histological picture of the pedicle of the lung separation. Parts of the wall of a large bronchus with ciliated epithelium, cartilage seen in the right half of the picture, bronchial glands on the lower rim, and a larger artery in the left half. H&E, × 125

The so-called pedicle in the area of the resection line consisted of a large bronchus with a wide lumen and containing blood vessels (Fig. 7).

Discussion

Different terms are used for the lung malformation consisting of abnormal arterial blood supply, bronchial anomalies and parenchymatous dysgenesis. The term "lung sequestration" is the one in most common use, although sequestration normally implies necrotic, dead tissue, which is not, however, the case in this malformation, whereas the term "separation" does characterize the nature of the condition.

Engelmann (1976), with his definition "lung malformation with abnormal haemodynamics", focuses attention clearly on the changed blood flow consistently associated with this anomaly. From the pathological viewpoint Tegtmeyer and Böhm (1984) prefer the main term "accessory lung", which can be subdivided into four different forms: (a) accessory lung lobe, (b) interlobar sequestration; (c) extralobar sequestration; and (d) bronchopulmonary malformation of the foregut.

For the clinician, the localization of the anomaly is important, and the names intra- and extralobar are insignificant, since both forms must be surgically removed. It must be questioned whether the whole range of preoperative investigations such as angiography, bronchography and upper GI X-ray series, is necessary. Practice suggests that this is not so. Five of our nine cases were incidental findings, and tumours had been suspected in three. Removal of the pathologic lung parts involved no technical difficulties.

There should be no connection with the tracheobronchial tree in extralobar forms. However, two cases have already been described in which such a connection did exist. On the basis of the pathohistological findings a communication with the tracheobronchial tree can be postulated in case 9 of Table 3, especially as a pedicle of the rounded, separated part ran paravertebrally and subpleurally in the direction of the tracheal bifurcation. The wide bronchi and relatively well unfolded alveoli seen in the histological preparations indicated ventilation that, while indeed not optimal, was adequate for unfolding, preventing mucus retention. Air entry via connections with the oesophagus is unlikely, since no inflammatory changes, food particles or gastric contents were found.

In 1985, Garstin et al. reported on three cases of extralobar separation with no signs of aeration. The pathologically changed lymph vessels within the separation in case 9 of Table 3 could reflect congenital angiectases. It is more probable, however, that they are secondary ectases induced by obstruction resulting from inadequate or even entirely deficient lymph drainage. The absence of larger lymph vessels in the pedicle supports this assumption. The recurrent unilateral pleural effusions effecting respiratory insufficiency by displacement could possibly be caused by chronic lymph obstruction. Thoracotomy was needed to clarify the diagnosis. The child recovered. A similar case with pleural effusion found on postmortem examination in a male premature newborn has been published by Tegtmeyer and Böhm (1984).

Acknowledgements. X-rays are reproduced by courtesy of the 1st Radiological Institute and the 2nd Radiological Institute of the Radiological Centre of the Klinikum Berlin-Buch.
CT scans were performed by the "Arbeitsgemeinschaft Ganzkörpercomputertomographie" of the Klinikum Berlin-Buch.

Summary

This paper refers to the different terminology used in so-called lung separation/ sequestration and to the standpoint of the pathologist. Theories of development are discussed. Clinical symptoms, diagnosis, indications for operation and operative technique are described, and nine cases of lung separation (six with extralobar and three with intralobar forms) tabulated analysed. Among them there is a 5-month-old female infant with extralobar lung separation in the right hemithorax resulting in recurrent pleural effusions with severe respiratory insufficiency. There was evidence of aeration in the pathohistological preparation. Pleural effusion and the origin of the aeration in the separated lung are discussed.

Résumé

Il est question des différents termes utilisés pour désigner la séparation ou séquestration pulmonaire et des conceptions des pathologistes. Les théories de l'évolution sont aussi discutées. On y décrit aussi les symptômes cliniques, le diagnostic, l'indication pour l'intervention, la technique opératoire et on analyse 9 cas de séquestration pulmonaire, deux formes extralobaires et trois formes intralobaires. Parmi ces cas, on insiste sur le cas d'une petite fille de cinq mois présentant une séquestration pulmonaire extralobaire avec épanchement pleural fréquent et insuffisance respiratoire grave. La préparation histologique indiquait une pneumatisation. Les auteurs discutent sur l'épanchement pleural et sur l'origine de l'injection aérienne dans ce segment pulmonaire séparé.

Zusammenfassung

In dem Beitrag wird auf die unterschiedliche Bezeichnung der sogenannten Lungenseparation-Lungensequestration hingewiesen und auch die Stellungnahme des Pathologen dazu angeführt. Entstehungstheorien sind angegeben. Symptome, Diagnostik, Operationsindikation und -technik werden besprochen und 9 Fälle, 6 extra-, 3 intralobäre Formen, tabellarisch analysiert. Darunter befindet sich ein 5 Monate alter weiblicher Säugling mit einer extralobären Separation im rechten Hemithorax, der zu rezidivierenden Pleuraergüssen mit schwerer Ateminsuffizienz führte. Das histologische Präparat hatte Zeichen einer Belüftung. Pleuraerguß und Ursprung der Luft in der Separation werden diskutiert.

References

Bettex M, Genton N, Stockmann M (1981) Kinderchirurgie. Thieme, Stuttgart
Boyden EA (1958) Bronchogenic cysts and the theory of intralobar sequestration: a new embryologic data. J Thorac Surg 35:604
Engelmann C (1976) Lungenfehlbildungen mit abnormer Hämodynamik. Z Erkrank Atmungsorgane 146:161
Garstin WIH, Potts SR, Boston VE (1985) Extra-lobar pulmonary sequestration. A report of three cases and a review of the literature with special reference to the embryogenesis. Z Kinderchir 60:104
Gebauer PW, Mason CB (1959) Intralobar pulmonary sequestration associated with anomalous pulmonary vessels. Dis Chest 30:282
Genton N (1981) In: Bettex M, Genton N, Stockmann M (eds) Kinderchirurgie. Thieme, Stuttgart, p 5.180
Gray SW, Skandalakis JE (1972) Cystic duplications of the trachea and bronchi. Sequestration of the lung. In: Embryology for surgeons. Saunders, Philadelphia
Halil KG, Kilman JW (1975) Pulmonary sequestration. J Thorac Cardiovasc Surg 70:928
Hasche E (1962) Die intralobäre Sequestration. Thoraxchirurgie 10:15
Herxheimer G (1901) Über einen Fall von echter Nebenlunge. Centralbl Pathol 12:529
Huber JJ (1777) Observationes aliquot de arteria singulari pulmoni consessa. Acta Helvet 8:85
Kaup J (1891) Zwei Fälle von Hernia diaphragmatica congenita mit Abtrennung eines Lungenteiles. Dissertation, Kiel

Krause I, Mau H (1972) Die Lungenseparation in Verbindung mit der Relaxatio diaphragmatica. Z Erkrank Atmungsorgane 137:215

Pryce DM (1946) Lower accessory pulmonary artery with intralobar sequestration of lung. A report of seven cases. J Pathol Bacteriol 58:475

Rektorzik E (1861) Über accessorische Lungenlappen. Wochenblatt der Zeitschr der KK Gesellschaft der Ärzte in Wien, XVIII. Jahrgang

Rokitansky S (1861) Lehrbuch der pathologischen Anatomie, vol II, p 44

Ruge E (1878) Demonstration in Gesellschaft für Geburtshilfe und Gynäkologie, Berlin. Berl Klin Wochenschr, p 401

Schwartz DL, So HB, Anban T, Greedon JJ (1983) Total lung sequestration in association with oesophageal arteria and multiple tracheo-oesophageal fistulae. Z Kinderchir 38:410

Smith RA (1975) Cited in Jona JZ, Raffensperger JG: Total sequestration of the right lung. J Thorac Cardiovasc Surg 69:361

Springer C (1898) Rudimentäre accessorische Lunge. Prag Med Wochenschr, p 393

Stöcker E (1972) Cited in Zwintz EF, Olbert F, Titscher R: Problematik und Diagnostik intralobärer Sequestration. Pneumologie 146:275

Tegtmeyer F, Böhm N (1984) Nebenlungen − Extralobäre Lungensequestration. Verh Dtsch Ges Pathol 68:476 / Fischer, Jena 1985

Voisin R (1903) Sur un cas de lobe erratique du poumon. Arch Med Expir Anat Pathol 15:228

Wimbish JJ, Agha FP, Brandy TM (1983) Bilateral pulmonary sequestration: computed tomographic appearance. AJR 140:689

Extralobar Sequestration of the Lung in Children

M. Leijala[1] and I. Louhimo[1]

Extralobar sequestration of the lung is defined as nonfunctioning lung tissue with no connection or only nonluminal connection with the normal bronchial tree, covered and surrounded by its own visceral pleura. This definition does not specify a blood supply from an anomalous systemic artery, which will be shown to be absent in many cases. Accessory lung, accessory lobe, pulmonary aberration, supernumerary lung, *Nebenlunge* and Rokitrasky lobe are here considered synonyms for extralobar sequestration.

The term sequestration was initially used by Price (1946), and since then extra- and intrapulmonary sequestration have commonly been described together. This may be misleading, because the typical forms are often quite different from a clinical point of view and the features of extralobar sequestration are easily obscured by the more common intralobar type. For example, in Carter's literature review (1969) of 228 cases of pulmonary sequestration there were only 30 cases of extralobar forms. In the largest series of extralobar sequestrations described in the literature (Oehlenschlaegel 1957; Savic et al. 1979) most cases were collected from autopsies, and this may also confuse the picture. Our own clinical experience with extralobar sequestration at least differs significantly from the textbook description of the condition.

We therefore describe the features of our 16 paediatric patients with extralobar sequestration of the lung. This is the largest series of patients with this disease to be reported from a single unit. All patients were clinically diagnosed and were operated upon. Special attention was given to the symptoms, blood supply, possible bronchial or oesophageal connection, and the presence of additional anomalies.

Patients

In 1961–1984, in all 38 patients with pulmonary sequestration were treated at the Children's Hospital belonging to the University of Helsinki, 22 of whom had intralobar sequestration only, 15 extralobar only, and 1 both types. Only the 16 patients with extralobar sequestrations are further analysed below. The age of the patients varied from 21 days to 12 years (mean 3.61 years); 6 were under 1 year

[1]Department of Paediatric Surgery, Children's Hospital, Helsinki University Central Hospital, Stenbäckinkatu 11, SF-00290 Helsinki, Finnland.

Progress in Pediatric Surgery, Vol. 21
Ed. by P. Wurnig
© Springer-Verlag Berlin Heidelberg 1987

and 12 under 5 years of age at the time of the operation. There were 11 boys and 5 girls. The sequestration was on the left side in 14 patients and on the right side in 3 patients. In contrast to many previous reports there were only seven left lower accessory lobes; the lesion was above the lung hilum in 7 cases and in the right lower pulmonary region in the remaining 2.

Symptoms

None of the patients had any cardiovascular symptoms, which is in accordance with the observation that systemic artery supply was often absent and was never provided by very large arteries. Most of the patients (12/16 = 75%) had some respiratory symptoms, the most common of which were: dyspnoea (9), pneumonia (5), coughing attacks (4), cyanosis (3), and asthmatic symptoms (2). The four patients without respiratory symptoms came to examination for other reasons: two because of funnel chest, one for abdominal symptoms, and one patient following a routine chest X-ray at school.

Preoperative Studies

Sequestration was seen on chest X-ray in all cases. Some of the roentgenological findings are presented in Fig. 1. With experience the picture of extralobar sequestration in the upper thorax was considered so typical that no other diagnostic procedure before the operation was performed. In the whole series angiography was carried out in six patients, which revealed large systemic arteries from the aorta in one case only. These arteries, however, went to the patient's simultaneous intralobar sequestration. In one other patient a small systemic artery from the aorta to the lung was seen. In two patients the angiography was slightly abnormal, showing an area of poor pulmonary vascularization. Preoperative bronchography was performed in six patients and showed distinct abnormality in only one, in whom there was a slight compression of the upper lobe bronchus.

Operative Findings

All 16 patients were operated on and the accessory lobe was removed. In two patients the left lower lobe was also excised, in one case because of lobar emphysema and in the other because of simultaneous intralobar sequestration. One patient also had an operation for his funnel chest.

Special attention was given to the blood supply of the accessory lung. In five patients the arterial blood came solely from the pulmonary artery. In four of these cases the sequestration was in the middle region of the thoracic cavity. The systemic artery came in two cases from the cervical arteries, in two cases from the aorta below the diaphragm and in seven cases from the thoracic aorta. The systemic arteries were never as large as in typical cases of intralobar sequestration, and in ten patients they were quite small or even rudimentary.

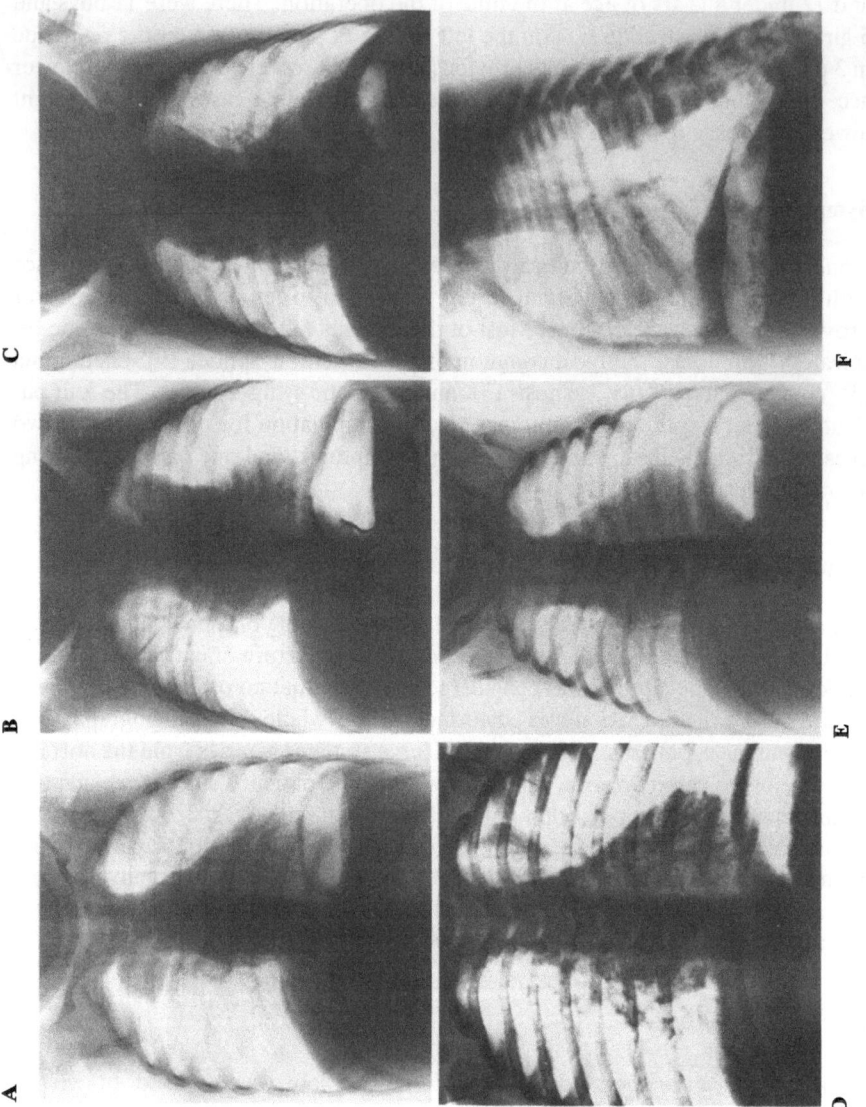

Fig. 1A–F. Chest X-ray findings in extralobar pulmonary sequestration. **A, B, D** upper accessory lobes; **C** left lower accessory lobe; **E, F**, two views of same posterior accessory lobe in midthorax

Venous return was to the pulmonary vein in eight and two systemic veins (vena azygos, hemiazygos or innominata), in eight cases.

Rudimentary bronchial remnants were found in six patients. This was connected to the oesophagus in one case and to the main bronchus or trachea in four; in one case there was a double trachea going towards the neck, where it ended in a cyst-like lesion (Fig. 2). This extra trachea had a definite lumen permitting intra-operative "bronchography".

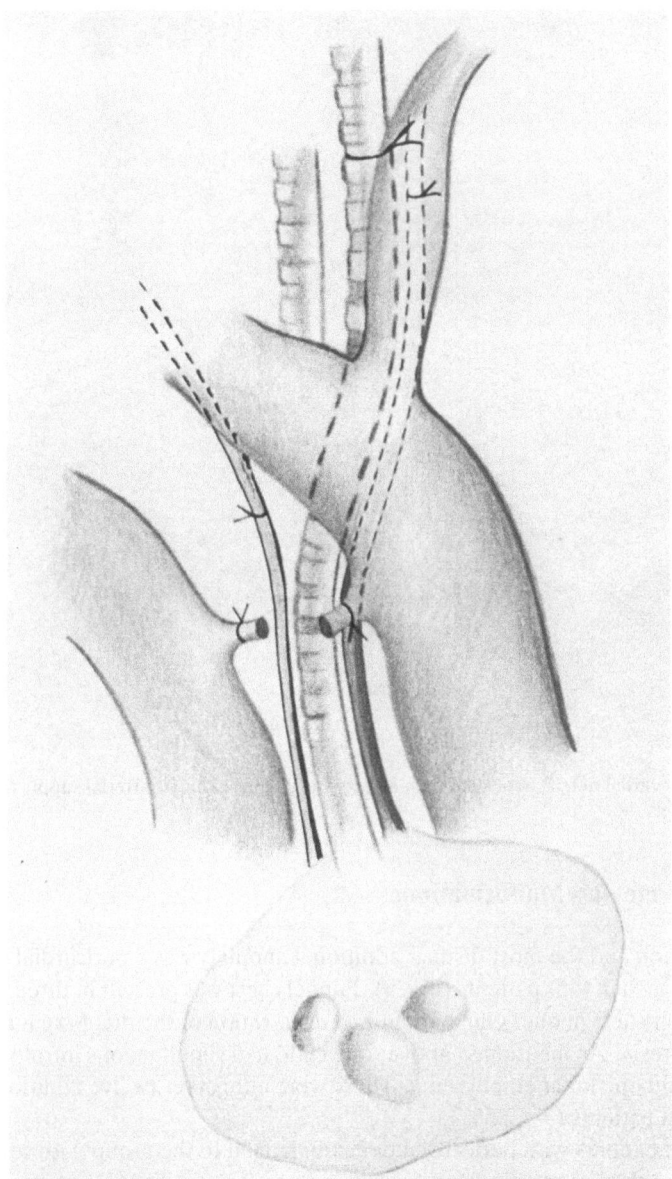

Fig. 2. Drawing of an accessory lobe with its own trachea

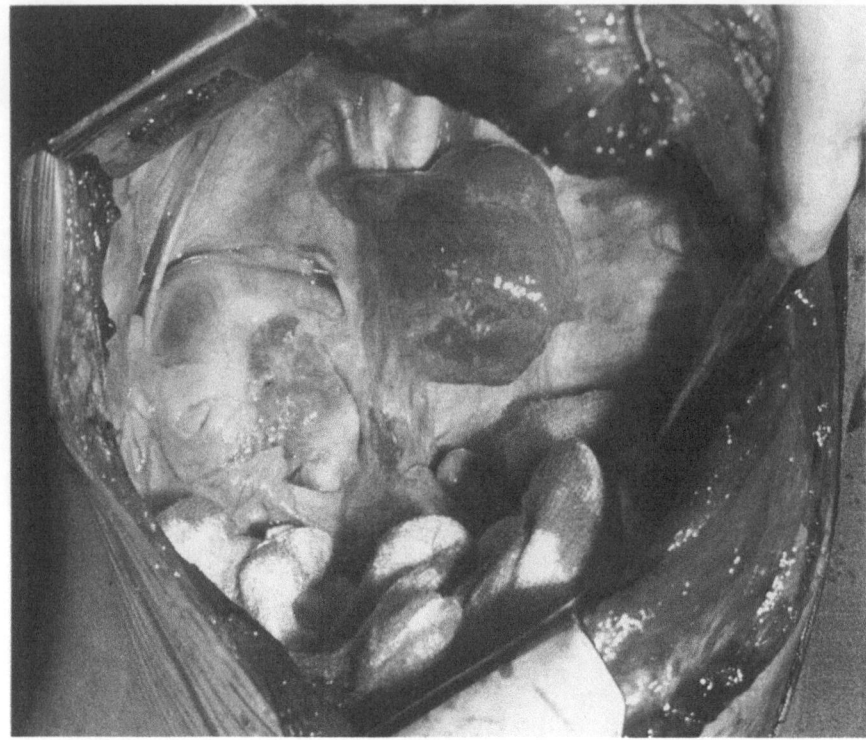

Fig. 3. A large pericardial defect associated with an accessory lobe having its arterial supply from the pulmonary artery

Additional Congenital Malformations

The most common and the most distinct additional anomaly was a pericardial defect, which was seen in four patients (Fig. 3). Funnel chest was present in three patients and pigeon chest in one. One patient had eventration of the diaphragm and one, choanal atresia. As mentioned above, one child had simultaneous intralobar sequestration and one lobar emphysema. There were altogether twelve additional anomalies in ten patients (= 62.5%).

Three of the patients with pericardial defect belonged to the group with some rudimentary bronchial connection.

Histology

Macroscopically all the accessory lungs were cystic, but all had definite lung tissue in addition, although mostly immature (Fig. 4). Bronchial epithelium, cartilage, and elastic or nonelastic arteries were also present. Bronchogenic cysts were excluded from this study.

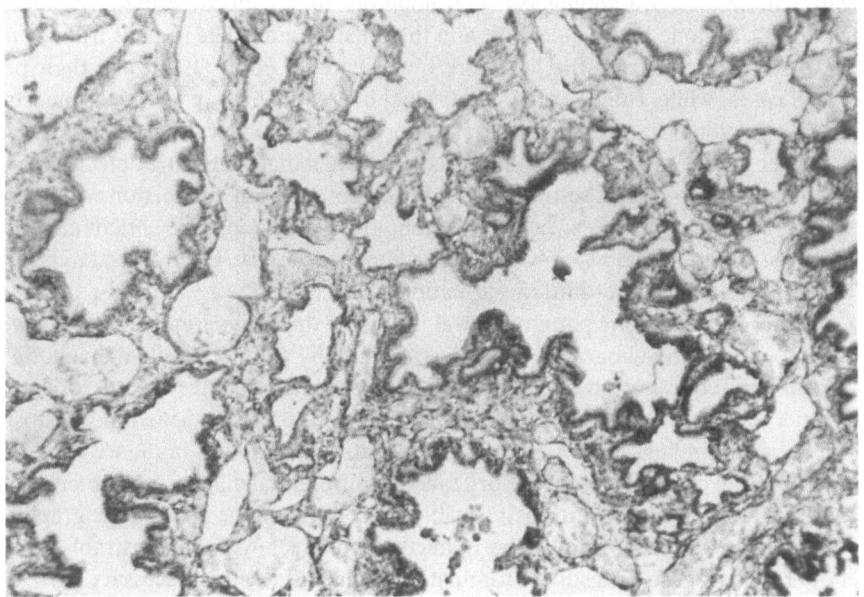

Fig. 4. A typical histological picture of an extrapulmonary sequestration

Discussion

The possible pathogenesis of pulmonary sequestration has been thoroughly discussed by various workers (Carter 1969; O'Mara et al. 1978; Sade et al. 1974). None of the theories can explain all the variants, which include systemic vascular supply of the lung without sequestration on the one end and extralobar sequestration with pulmonary vascular supply on the other. The so-called vascular theories (Price 1946; Smith 1956) obviously do not explain the many cases were the systemic vessels are not present. Our patient with double trachea excludes any primary vascular aetiology, and the simultaneous occurrence of pericardial defects also makes this unlikely.

Ectopic budding from the primitive foregut is an obvious explanation for our cases of extralobar sequestration, but the origin of the large anomalous vessels supplying normal lung remains obscure, as does that of pericardial defect. Still, the presence of both extra- and intralobar sequestration in the same patient and the fact that all possible transitional forms of typical intra- to typical extralobar sequestration have been described support a common aetiology of both types (Blesovsky 1967; Gerle et al. 1968).

In our series the clinical picture deviates considerably from that reported in textbooks and papers in the American literature, where the extralobar type of sequestration is still often described as a lower accessory lobe which occurs simultaneously with diaphragmatic defect in 60%–80% of cases (Canthy 1981; Kendig and Chermic 1983; Landing 1979). Among the 10 patients described by Buntain et al. (1979) none had sequestration in the upper thorax. The same is true for the 24 cases collected from the literature by de Paredes et al. (1970) and their personal cases, while Tumbro et al. (1975) had one patient of six with the sequestration in the upper thorax. In our series upper accessory lobe was almost as common as lower accessory lobe, and in no case was there a diaphragmatic defect.

A pericardial defect, although previously described in connection with extralobar sequestration, was seen more commonly in our series (25%) than in earlier reports. Arterial blood supply from the pulmonary artery, often considered rare, was seen in almost one-third of our patients.

From the diagnostic point of view it is notable that angiography rarely allowed diagnosis and bronchography never. Arteriography allows definitive diagnosis in intralobar requestration, but not in accessory lung. In typical cases of upper thorax sequestration arteriography is now not routinely performed in our hospital. Normal findings do not exclude sequestration and do not influence the treatment. In the case of lower accessory lobe the differential diagnosis between extra- and intralobar sequestration is probably more safely done when angiography is performed. Connection to the oesophagus or stomach with demonstrable lumen is so rare that gastrointestinal examinations are considered unnecessary.

Most of the patients were, a little surprisingly, symptomatic, which indicates the necessity of surgical treatment. An extralobar sequestration is more easily excised than an intralobar sequestration, as no normal lung tissue is removed and the operation is not dangerous. Following removal of the lesion the diagnosis can be confirmed, and excision is therefore recommended for this reason also. Some forms of bronchogenic cysts that extend into the pleural cavity cannot be distinguished from pulmonary sequestration except by histological examination. Any pericardial defect may need surgical attention: in one patient the left atrial appendix was amputated to prevent it from becoming incarcerated in the pericardial cavity.

In summary, the clinical picture of extralobar sequestration varies considerably and many of the "typical" features, such as systemic arterial supply, left lower lobe localization and diaphragmatic defect, are often absent. With experience, diagnosis and treatment are easy.

Summary

Sixteen patients with extralobar sequestration of the lung are reported on. The age at time of diagnosis varied from 21 days to 12 years (mean 3.6 years). Most of the patients presented with respiratory symptoms, such as dyspnoea, pneumonia, coughing attacks, cyanosis and asthmatic symptoms, but diagnosis was made incidentally in 4. Diagnosis was established by chest X-ray in every case. Preoperative angiography and bronchography was carried out in six cases. All 16 patients underwent thoracotomy for removal of the sequestration. Rudimentary bronchial remnants were found in 6 cases. Extralobar sequestration was associated with 12 additional malformations in 10 of the 16 patients. The clinical picture varies considerably and many of the "typical" features, such as systemic arterial blood supply, left lower lobe localization and diaphragmatic defect, are often absent. Diagnosis and treatment are easy.

Résumé

Il est question de l'observation de 16 cas de séquestration pulmonaires extralobaires. Les patients sont âgés de 21 jours à 12 ans (3 ans et demi en moyenne). La plupart des patients présentent des symptômes respiratoires tels que dyspnée, pneumonie, crises de toux, cyanose et symptômes asthmatiques. Dans 4 cas, il s'agit d'un diagnostic fortuit. Dans tous les cas, une radiographie du thorax a été à l'origine du diagnostic. Dans six cas, on procéda à une angiographie et à une bronchographie avant l'intervention. Tous les patients subirent une thoracotomie pour remédier à la séquestration. Dans six des cas, on trouva des résidus bronchiaux rudimentaires. Dix des seize patients présentaient en outre douze autres malformations. Les symptômes cliniques sont très variés et souvent, on ne rencontre pas les signes "caractéristiques" tels qu'irrigation sanguine systémique, localisation au niveau du lobe gauche inférieur et défaut au niveau du diaphragme. Le diagnostic et la thérapeutique ne présentent pas de difficultés.

Zusammenfassung

Es wird über 16 Patienten mit extralobärer Lungensequestration berichtet. Das Alter bei Diagnosestellung variierte von 21 Tagen bis 12 Jahre (im Mittel 3,6 Jahre). Die meisten der Patienten zeigten respiratorische Probleme wie Dyspnoe, Pneumonie, Hustenattacken, Zyanose and asthmatische Symptome, wogegen es sich 4mal um Zufallsbefunde handelte. Die Diagnose wurde durch Thoraxaufnahmen bei allen Fällen gestellt. Sechsmal wurde eine präoperative Angiographie und Bronchographie durchgeführt. Alle 16 Patienten wurden zur Entfernung der Lungensequestration thorakotomiert. Zehn der 16 Patienten hatten 12 begleitende Fehlbildungen. Rudimentäre Bronchialanteile wurden 6mal gefunden. Das klinische Bild der extralobären Sequestration variiert beträchtlich, und oft fehlen „typische" Zeichen wie systemische arterielle Blutversorgung, Lokalisation im linken Unterlappen und Zwerchfelldefekte. Diagnose und Behandlung sind einfach.

References

Blesovsky A (1967) Pulmonary sequestration. A report of an unusual case and a review of the literature. Thorax 22:351–357
Buntain WL, Woolley MM, Mahour GH, Isaacs H, Payne V (1977) Pulmonary sequestration in children: A twenty-five year experience. Surgery 81:413–420

Canthy TG (1981) Extralobar pulmonary sequestration. Unusual presentation and systemic vascular communication in association with a right sided diaphragmatic hernia. J Thorac Cardiovasc Surg 81:96–99

Carter R (1969) Pulmonary sequestration. Ann Thorac Surg 7:68–88

De Parades CG, Pierce WS, Johnson DG, Waldhausen JA (1979) Pulmonary sequestration in infants and children: a 20-year experience and review of the literature. J Pediatr Surg 5:136–147

Gerle RD, Jaretzki A, Ashley CA, Berne AS (1968) Congenital bronchopulmonary-foregut malformation. Pulmonary sequestration communicating with the gastrointestinal tract. N Engl J Med 278:1413–1419

Kendig EL Jr, Chernick V (1983) Disorders of the respiratory tract in children, 4th edn. Saunders, Philadelphia

Landing BH (1979) Congenital malformations and genetic disorders of the respiratory tract. Am Rev Respir Dis 120:151–185

Oehlschlaegel G (1957) Zur Systematik und Pathogenese der Nebenlungen. Frankfurter Zeitschrift für Pathologie 68:71–85

O'Mara CS, Baker RR, Jeysingham K (1978) Pulmonary sequestration. Surg Gynecol Obstet 147:609–616

Pryce DM (1946) Lower accessory pulmonary artery with intralobar sequestration of lung. J Pathol (Lond) 58:457–467

Sade RM, Clouse M, Ellis FH (1974) The spectrum of pulmonary sequestration. Ann Thorac Surg 18:644–658

Savic B, Birtel FJ, Tholen W, Funke HD, Knoche R (1979) Lung sequestration: report of seven cases and review of 540 published cases. Thorax 34:96–101

Smith RA (1956) A theory of the origin of intralobar sequestration of lung. Thorax 11:10–24

Zumbro GL, Seitter G, Strevey TE, Green DC (1975) Pulmonary sequestration: a broad spectrum of bronchopulmonary foregut abnormalities. Ann Thorac Surg 20:161–169

Scimitar Syndrome
and Associated Pulmonary Sequestration:
Report of a Successfully Corrected Case

E. Horcher[1] and F. Helmer[1]

Introduction

The scimitar syndrome is characterized by anomalous venous drainage from the right lung to the vena cava inferior. The appearance of this vein on chest X-ray is suggestive of a Turkish sword and is called the "scimitar" sign by Neill et al. (1960). The condition may be associated with anomalies of the right lung (absence of lung fissures, mirror image of the left lung, absence of lobe bronchi), anomalies of the pulmonary artery, and congenital heart defects (Mathey et al. 1968; Mende et al. 1973). The symptoms are similar to those of an atrial septal defect due to a left-to-right shunt, such as repeated respiratory infections. We present an uncommon case of scimitar syndrome combined with pulmonary sequestration; few cases of this anomaly have been reported in the literature (Alivizatos et al. 1985; Ohsaki 1983).

Case Report

A 6-month-old boy was transferred from Libya to our clinic because of recurrent pulmonary infections and effort dyspnoea. Chest X-ray led us to suspect atelectasis of the right lower lobe; a scimitar vein was not recognized at this point (Fig. 1). Bronchoscopy showed a normal bronchial tree without obstruction, but the middle lobe bronchus could not be identified. In echocardiography dilatation of both ventricles was found but no atrial or ventricular septum defect, and valve function was normal. The pulmonary veins were recognized only on the left side. Cardiac catheterization demonstrated a left-to-right shunt of 23% and atypical branching of the right pulmonary artery with absence of a pulmonary arterial supply to the right lower lobe (Fig. 2).

The venous phase of the pulmonary angiogram showed an atypical common pulmonary vein descending along the right side of the heart and draining nearly all the blood from the right lung into the vena cava inferior. Only a minor lung vein from the upper lobe seemed to drain into the left atrium (Fig. 3). The aortogram showed two systemic arteries arising from the abdominal aorta, supplying the right lower lobe of the lung (Fig. 4). The diagnosis of a scimitar vein and pulmonary sequestration was made. The pressure in the pulmonary artery was 35/12/

[1]Department of Pediatric Surgery, Second Surgical University Clinic, A-1090 Vienna, Austria

Progress in Pediatric Surgery, Vol. 21
Ed. by P. Wurnig
© Springer-Verlag Berlin Heidelberg 1987

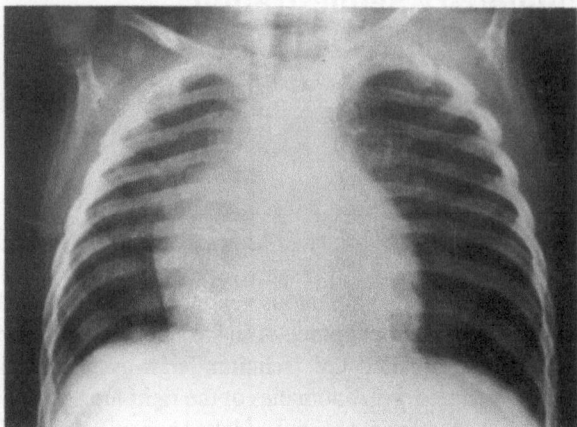

Fig. 1. On the chest X-ray the scimitar vein is hardly distinguishable from the right cardiac border owing to dextrocardia

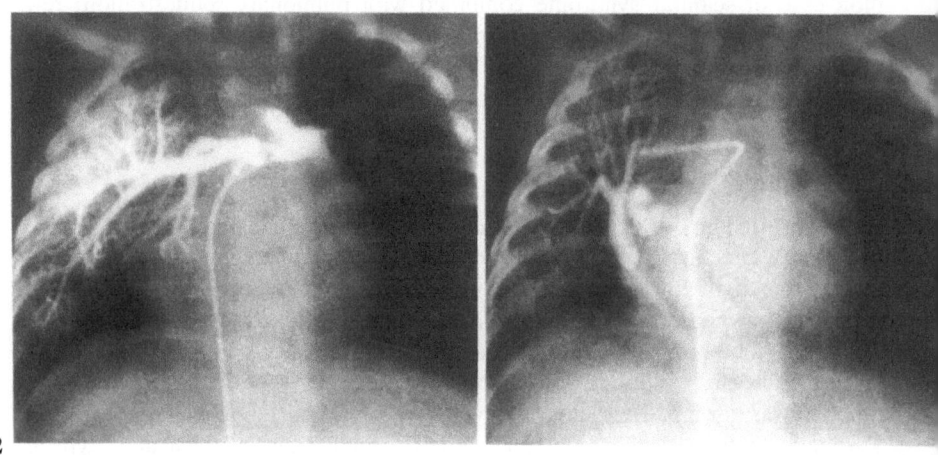

2

Fig. 2. Pulmonary arteriogram showing absence of pulmonary artery supply to the right lower lobe

Fig. 3. Venous phase of the pulmonary arteriogram showing the scimitar vein along the right cardiac border and a tortuous vein entering the left atrium

18 mm Hg, and systemic pressure was 75/30/50 mm Hg. Figure 5 shows the entire anomaly.

At operation the right pleural space was found to be partly obliterated by adhesions. The right lung showed no interlobar segmentation. As seen in the angiogram, a large anomalous venous trunk descended in a sulcus of the lower lobe along the right heart and drained the veins from the entire right lung into the

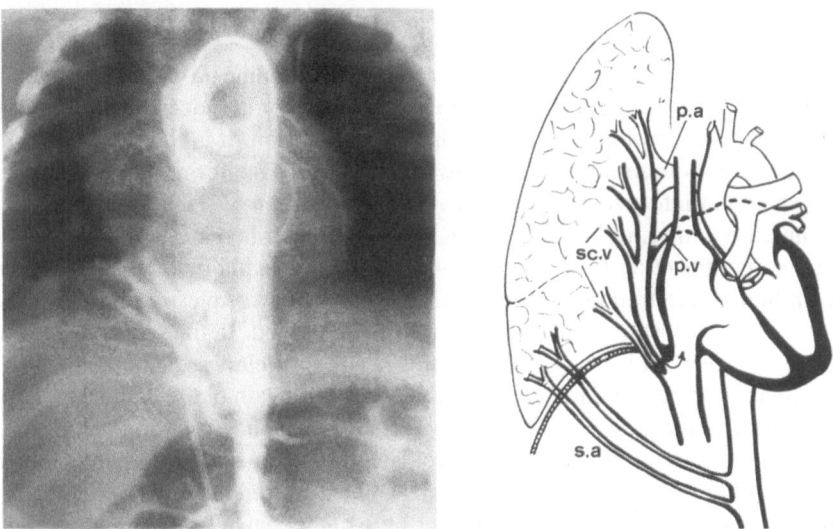

Fig. 4. Aortogram: two systemic arteries from the abdominal aorta supply the sequestrated right lower lobe

Fig. 5. Diagram of the vascular anomalies of the right lung showing hypoplastic pulmonary artery *(p.a.)*, Scimitar vein *(sc.v.)*, two systemic arteries *(s.a.)* and pulmonary vein from lower lobe *(p.v.)*

infradiaphragmatic vena cava inferior. One systemic artery 5 mm in diameter entered the diaphragm in a dorsolateral position, and another one, 3 mm in diameter, in a more ventral and medial position.

In a first step all vessels at the hilus were isolated, beginning with the pulmonary artery, and an apparent normal pulmonary vein was then found. The two diaphragmatic arteries were ligated. Then the scimitar vein was freed from the sulcus in the lower lobe and the diaphragm. A small vein from the sequestrated lobe was descending through the diaphragm collateral to the scimitar vein and was ligated at the vena cava inferior. Further preparation demonstrated that the minor lung vein, which seemed to drain the upper lobe, arose from the sequestrated lobe and drained into the left atrium. This vein was also ligated. The sequestrated lobe therefore had venous drainage into the left atrium as well as into the vena cava inferior. After preparation of all the vessels the lower lobe bronchus was dissected and the demarcation line between the normal and the sequestrated parenchyma of the unlobulated lung became visible and the sequestrated lower lobe was resected. The middle lobe was rudimentary. The scimitar vein was excised with a circular flap from the vena cava inferior and easily reanastomosed to the left atrium end-to-side with a 6.0 PDS continuous suture using a side occluding clamp with no need for extracorporeal circulation. The postoperative course was uneventful except for pleural effusions which required pleurocentesis.

Discussion

The scimitar syndrome is usually an incidental finding in children or adults. Whether or not an operation is necessary depends on the degree of left-to-right shunt and the development of pulmonary hypertension. It is advisable to resect a pulmonary sequestration as soon as the diagnosis is confirmed, because of the possibility of infective complications. The combination of scimitar syndrome and pulmonary sequestration is rare. Ohsaki (1983) described a case similar to ours, and Alivizatos et al. (1985) found this condition in 2 children among 12 patients with lung sequestrations. In one of these children the sequestrated lobe was resected and correction of the scimitar syndrome delayed. In the second patient the anomaly was not recognized preoperatively and the vein was ligated, resulting in acute haemorrhagic infarction of the right lung and death of the patient. Accurate preoperative diagnosis by cardiac catheterization is mandatory for selection of the appropriate surgical procedure and avoidance of fatal mistakes. Physiological correction of the pulmonary venous return can be achieved by direct anastomosis of the simitar vein in appropriate cases or by a tunnel patch or a conduit (Hallman and Cooley 1975; Lichea and Ursinus 1983). In the literature (Alivizatos et al. 1985) a two-stage procedure is suggested for this anomaly. Total correction in a one-stage intervention was easily achieved in our case, however. The disadvantage of a rather small anastomosis in a baby was offset by excising part of the vena cava inferior to widen the anastomosis and by using a resorbable monofil suture material in anticipation of future growth of the anastomosis.

Summary

A case of scimitar syndrome with pulmonary sequestration is reported. Anomalous pulmonary venous return from the right lung to the infradiaphragmatic vena cava inferior was diagnosed by pulmonary angiogram and sequestration of the right lower lobe was confirmed by aortogram. Venous return from the sequestrated lung was partly into the vena cava inferior and partly into the left atrium. Successful repair was achieved by resection of the sequestrated lobe and direct reimplantation of the scimitar vein into the left atrium. Accurate preoperative diagnosis and intraoperative evaluation of the anatomy is mandatory to correct this rare anomaly.

Résumé

Observation d'un cas de syndrome du cimeterre avec séquestration pulmonaire. Reflux veineux anormal du poumon droit dans la veine cave inférieure infradiaphragmatique, diagnostic par angiographie pulmonaire et séquestration du lobe inférieur droit confirmé par aortographie. Reflux veineux du poumon séquestré en partie dans la veine cave inférieure et en partie dans l'atrium gauche.

Nous avons pratiqué avec succès une résection du lobe séquestré et une réimplantation directe de la veine cimeterre dans l'atrium gauche. Un diagnostic préopératoire d'une grande précision et un examen minutieux des conditions anatomiques durant l'intervention sont absolûment nécessaires pour pouvoir corriger cette anomalie rare.

Zusammenfassung

Es wird über einen Fall von Scimitar-Syndrom mit Lungensequestration berichtet. Ein abnormer pulmonaler venöser Rückstrom von der rechten Lunge in die infradiaphragmatische Vena cava wurde durch die Pulmonalangiographie diagnostiziert und die Sequestration des rechten Unterlappens durch die Aortographie bestätigt. Der venöse Rückstrom aus dem sequestrierten Lungenteil erfolgte teils in die Vena cava inferior, teils in den linken Vorhof. Die erfolgreiche Korrektur erfolgte durch die Resektion des sequestrierten Lappens und die direkte Einpflanzung der Scimitarvene in den linken Vorhof. Eine exakte präoperative Diagnostik und intraoperative Klärung der anatomischen Verhältnisse ist zwingend notwendig, um diese seltene Anomalie erfolgreich zu korrigieren.

References

Alivizatos P, Cheatle T, de Leval M, Stark J (1985) Pulmonary sequestration complicated by anomalies of pulmonary venous return. J Pediatr Surg 20:76–79

Hallman GL, Cooley DA (1975) Surgical treatment of congenital heart disease, 2nd edn. Lea and Febiger, Philadelphia, pp 194–196

Lichea C. Ursinus W (1983) Die operative Behandlung des Scimitarsyndroms. Zentralbl Chir 108:159–166

Mathey J, Galey JJ, Logeais Y, et al (1968) Anomalous pulmonary venous return into inferior vena cava and associated bronchovascular anomalies (the scimitar syndrome). Thorax 23:398–407

Mende S, Kallfelz HC, Kreutzberg B (1973) Scimitar-Syndrom. Pathologie, Klinik und Therapie. Klin Padiatr 185:421–436

Neill CA, Ferenca C, Sabiston DC, Shelton J (1960) The familial occurrence of hypoplastic right lung with systemic arterial supply and venous drainage: Scimitar syndrome. John Hopkins Med J 107:1–20

Ohsaki Y (1983) Case of scimitar syndrome with pulmonary sequestration. Nippon Kyobu Shikkan Gakkai Zasshi 21:904–909

Congenital Cystic Adenomatoid Malformation of the Lung

M. R. Becker[1], F. Schindera[2], and W. A. Maier[1]

Introduction

At first, congenital cystic adenomatoid malformation (CCAM) of the lung can only be a clinical suspicion to be checked out in any differential diagnosis concerned with lung cysts. Only precise histomorphological examination renders diagnosis possible. In 1949, Ch'in and Tang described such a lung malformation, which was associated with generalized anasarca (skin oedema) and hydramnion.

Wexler and Dapena (1978) presented 200 cases collected from the literature. Diagnosis was established during the first year of life in 90% of the children.

Table 1. Histological classification of congenital cystic adenomatoid malformation of pulmonary CCAM (Stocker et al. 1977)

Type	Cyst size	Wall structure					Remarks
		Epithelium	Smooth muscle	Con-nec-tive tissue	Elastic fibres	Cartilage	
I	>1 cm	Ciliated	Present	Loose	Present	Very little	Alveolus-like structures and small cysts between large cysts
II	<1 cm	Cylindrical to cuboid	Irregular smooth muscle bundles	Loose	Tight elastic fibre network	Only as normal component of bronchi	Thin cyst wall
III	<0.5 cm	Cuboid	Some, isolated	Loose	Few	Absent	Similarity with glandoid structure of fetal lung, mostly whole lobe affected

[1]Paediatric Surgical Clinic and [2]Paediatric Clinic, Städtisches Klinikum Karlsruhe, D-7500 Karlsruhe, FRG.

Progress in Pediatric Surgery, Vol. 21
Ed. by P. Wurnig
© Springer-Verlag Berlin Heidelberg 1987

Classification of CCAM initially caused some difficulty, since CCAM was regarded by some as a kind of pulmonary sequestration, and by others, as lung cysts, lobar emphysema or simply hamartomas, as described by Albrechts (Stocker and Kagan-Hallett 1977; Stocker et al. 1978). According to Stocker et al. (1978), CCAM can be classified histologically into three types; for this purpose importance attaches to size and content and to the structure and consistency of the wall. All three types have in common an increase of adenomatoid structures similar to terminal bronchioli, cysts lined with cuboid or cylindrical epithelium and, finally, an increased amount of elastic connective tissue and absence of any inflammatory changes (Table 1).

Other authors, such as Östör et al. (1978), consider that Stocker's type III is the only really adenomatoid type, and associate type II with congenital lung cysts. Bale (1979) also regards the cystic structures as a malformation of the bronchioli and is of the opinion that CCAM is only a particular variant of so-called congenital cystic disease. It is certain that a localized maturation disturbance of lung tissue is present.

Embryologically, type I, with the highest degree of differentiation, is believed to develop at some time up to the 10th week of gestation and type II up to the 5th week, whereas type III, with the lowest degree of differentiation, is referred to days 26–28 of gestation. The aetiology of this malformation remains unclear so far.

In the majority of publications the congenital anomaly is described as unilateral, sometimes in a whole lobe or a part of it or in segments. Clinical symptoms vary according to the extension: dyspnoea and tachypnoea are the most prominent, progressing in some cases to acute respiratory distress syndrome with overinflation of the affected lung and mediastinal displacement. Development of a tension pneumothorax has also repeatedly been reported (Gaisie and Sang 1983). If the condition is not treated surgically, pulmonary infections and recurrent pneumonia result. The chest X-ray picture is not necessarily pathognomonic:

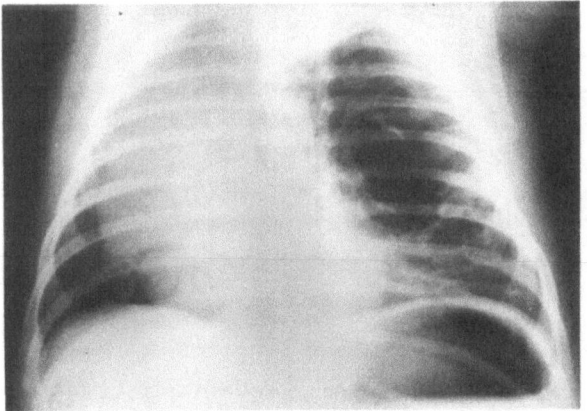

Fig. 1. Large area of cystic shadowing in left upper lobe with rightward mediastinal displacement

multiple round shadows with striated patterns may be seen, and a large cyst may mimic a pneumothorax following overinflation. However, real tension pneumothorax with mediastinal displacement during artificial ventilation may also develop. The following clinical entities must be included in the differential diagnosis: lung cysts, lung sequestration with cystic changes, lobar emphysema and diaphragmatic hernia.

An inquiry of ten paediatric surgical hospitals in the Federal Republic of Germany brought out how rare this malformation is. A 4-week-old infant underwent resection of the left upper lobe for lobar emphysema at the Paediatric surgical clinic of the University of Tübingen (Fig. 1). Pathohistological examination revealed type I CCAM. Another histologically confirmed case of CCAM has been reported from the paediatric surgical clinic of the Hospital in Schwabing, Munich.

Case Report

The case discussed in this paper was observed in a mature male newborn who developed cyanosis 4 h after birth. He presented with nose vibrations, alternating respiration and peripheral cyanosis. Chest X-ray revealed nearly homogeneous shadowing extending over 5–6 cm of the right middle and lower pulmonary fields and mediastinal displacement to the left (Fig. 2). Sonography revealed a spherical

Figs. 2–5. Course in subject of case report

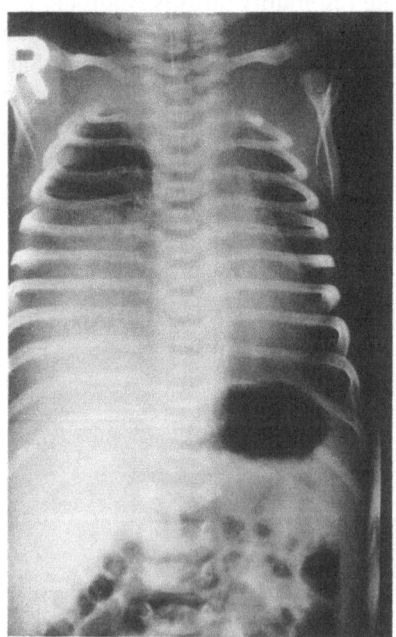

Fig. 2. Preoperative X-ray

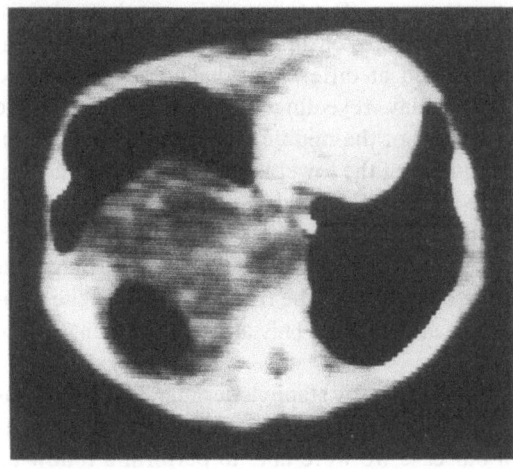

Fig. 3. CT scan of malformation

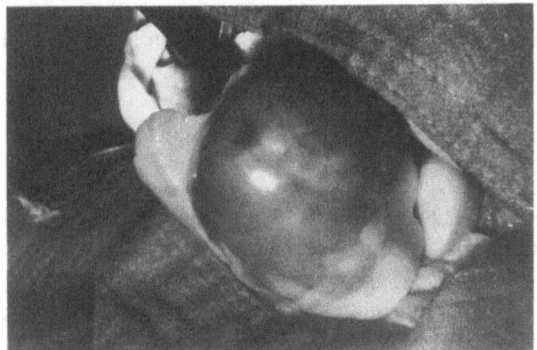

Fig. 4. Intraoperative view of malformation

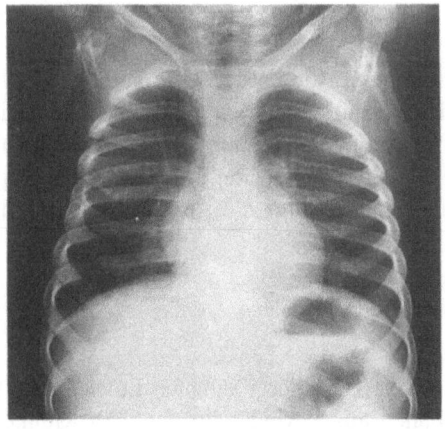

Fig. 5. Follow-up chest X-ray 2 years after surgery

tumour 6 cm in diameter with cystic structures. The CT scan (Fig. 3) showed a displacing process with loculated, aerated cavities of different size. Lung sequestration was one of the conditions suspected at differential diagnosis. Right-sided thoracotomy was carried out on the 4th day, revealing a first-sized tumour in the right lower lobe extending to the borders of the middle and upper lobes (Fig. 4). It originated from the laterobasal segment of the lower lobe. Enucleation and segmental resection with closure of the segmental bronchi were carried out. Pathohistological examination revealed cystic structures less than 1 cm in diameter, lined with partly cuboid and partly cylindrical epithelium. Neither cartilaginous parts nor inflammatory infiltrations were present. The transition zone to the adjacent lung tissue showed compression atelectases. This allowed confirmation of type-II CCAM could be confirmed.

The postoperative course was complicated by staphylodermia. The infant was discharged from hospital 4 weeks postoperatively. All three infants reported overcame the operation very well. In our case we were able to perform a follow-up examination 2 years after successful operation and found the child in a perfect healthy condition. The follow-up chest X-ray showed a normal central position of the heart and mediastinum (Fig. 5).

Basically, the prognosis of CCAM is good if it is diagnosed in good time and treated adequately.

Summary

The clinical and pathologic-anatomical picture of this rare lung malformation is described with reference to three cases from three different paediatric surgical hospitals. Methods of differential diagnosis against lung sequestration, pulmonary cysts, lobar emphysema, diaphragmatic hernia and pneumothorax are indicated. A definitive diagnosis and classification can be made only by means of histomorphological examinations.

Résumé

Les aspects cliniques et anatomo-pathologiques de cette malformation rare du poumon sont décrits sur la base de trois cas, traits dans trois cliniques de chirurgie infantile. On y traite du diagnostic différentiel et de l'analyse de la séquestration du poumon, des kystes pulmonaires, de l'emphysème lobaire, de la hernie diaphragmatique et du pneumothorax. Le diagnostic définitif n'est possible qu'à l'aide d' examens histo-morphologiques.

Zusammenfassung

Das klinische und pathologisch-anatomische Bild dieser seltenen Lungenfehlbildung wird im Zusammenhang mit 3 Fällen aus 3 Kinderchirurgischen Kliniken dargestellt. Auf die differentialdiagnostische Abgrenzung gegenüber der Lungensequestration, der Lungenzyste, dem lobären Emphysem sowie gegenüber der Zwerchfellhernie und dem Pneumothorax wird hingewiesen. Die endgültige Diagnose und Klassifikation ist nur aufgrund histomorphologischer Untersuchungen zu stellen.

References

Bale PM (1979) Congenital cystic malformation of the lung. A form of congenital bronchiolar ("adenomatoid") malformation. Am J Clin Pathol 71:411

Ch'in KY, Tang MY (1949) Congenital adenomatoid malformation of one lobe of a lung with general anasarca. Arch Pathol 48:221

Gaisie G, Sang-oh K (1983) Spontaneous pneumothorax in cystic adenomatoid malformation. Pediatr Radiol 13:281

Östör AG, Stillwell R, Fortune DW (1978) Bilateral pulmonary agenesis. Pathology 10:243

Stocker JT, Kagan-Hallet K (1977) Congenital cystic adenomatoid malformation of the lung. Classification and morphologic spectrum. Hum Pathol 8:155

Stocker JT, Drake RM, Madewell JE (1978) Cystic and congenital lung disease in newborns. In: Rosenberg HS, Bolande RP (eds) Perspectives in pediatric pathology, vol 4. Yearbook Med Publ, Chicago, p 93

Wexler HA, Dapena MV (1978) Congenital cystic adenomatoid malformation. Radiology 26:737

Experience in Surgical Treatment
of Pulmonary and Bronchial Tumours in Childhood

W. Tischer[2], H. Reddemann[5], P. Herzog[2], K. Gdanietz[1], J. Witt[3], P. Wurnig[3], and A. Reiner[4]

Introduction

Tumours of the lungs and bronchi in childhood are so rare that Marsden and Scholtz (1976) observed only four lung tumours among 2207 malignancies in children over a 20-year period. Only isolated cases have been dealt with in most reports so far. It therefore seemed useful to attempt a review showing how many and what types of lung tumours in children were observed at different paediatric surgical centres over a fairly long time.

This report summarizes the cases observed at the Paediatric Surgical clinics of Berlin-Buch and Greifswald in the German Democratic Republic and at the Department of Paediatric Surgery of the Mautner Markhof Children's Hospital in Vienna from 1963 to 1983.

The patients of the Paediatric Surgical Hospitals in Leipzig, German Democratic Republic, and Zurich, Switzerland, have been reported in the literature but are also included (Meissner et al. 1976; Stauffer 1982).* Table 1 reviews all the cases of lung and bronchial tumours. Four children had lung malignancies; three of these died and one was cured. Tumour enucleation and nonradical tumour extirpation were each performed in one case, while lobectomy and segmental resection were each performed in one of the remaining two cases. Selected cases are briefly reported.

Case 1

Boy, date of birth 9 September 1973

Anamnesis: "Illness" for 4 weeks when he was 5 years old in 1978 subfebrile temperature, tiredness, vomiting, coughing, poor general condition.

---

* Cordial thanks to Prof. F. Meissner of Leipzig and Prof. U. Stauffer of Zurich who placed the cases of Table 2 and 3 at our's disposal.

[1] Paediatric Surgical Clinic, Karowerstraße 10, DDR-1115 Berlin-Buch, GDR.
[2] Paediatric Surgical Clinic, DDR-2200 Greifswald, GDR.
[3] Surgical Department of the Mautner Markhof Children's Hospital, Baumgasse 75, A-1030 Vienna, Austria.
[4] Institute of Pathological Anatomy, University of Vienna, Spitalgasse 4, A-1090 Vienna, Austria.
[5] Pediatric University Clinic Greifswald, DDR-2200 Greifswald, GDR.

Table 1. Review of the cases treated at the Paediatric Surgical Clinics in Greifswald and Berlin-Buch (GDR) and the Department of Paediatric Surgery of the Mautner Markhof Kinderspital in Vienna (Austria)

Pat. no.	Age	Sex	Anamnesis	Histology	Site	Treatment	Chemo-therapy	Outcome
1	4.5 years	m	Tiredness, coughing and fever for 4 weeks	Pulmonary embryoma	Left lung	Nonradical tumour excision; repeat thoracotomy 10 months later for recurrence	+	Death 13 months later
2	5 years	m	Coughing, sepsis, lung cysts	Pulmonary embryoma	Right lower lobe	Right lower lobectomy	+	Death 17 months later
3	11 years	f	Coughing, weight loss	Malignant papillomatous pleural meso-thelioma	Left lower lobe	Enucleation + radiation therapy		Cured
4	1.5 years	m	Bronchitis, incidental finding	Fibrous reticulo-sarcoma in a hamartoma	Right lower lobe	Segmental resection	+	Death 14 months later
5	24 h	m	Cyanosis, dextrocardia, suspected diaphragmatic hernia	Hamartoma, alveolar dys-plasia, CCAM	Left upper lobe	Lobectomy following laparotomy		Death
6	6 months	f	Pneumonia	Cystic hamartoma, CCAM	Right upper lobe	Lobectomy		Well

Table 1 (continued)

Pat. no.	Age	Sex	Anamnesis	Histology	Site	Treatment	Chemo-therapy	Outcome
7	24 h	m	Cyanosis, thoracic wall retractions	Hamartoma, CCAM	Right lower lobe	Lobectomy		Well
8	11 years	m	Incidental finding, round focus	Hamartoma	Left lower lobe	Lobectomy		Well
9	3 years	m	Cyanosis, r-l-shunt, drumstick fingers	Arteriovenous angioma	Right lower lobe	Lobectomy		Well
10	12 years	f	Coughing, recurrent pneumonia for 1 year	Mucoepidermoid tumour	Right middle lobe	Bilobectomy		Free of recurrence for 5 years
11	8 years	m	Recurrent pneumonia	Malignant mucoepidermoid tumour	Left main bronchus	Circumferential resection		Free of recurrence for 6 years
12	8 years	f	Recurrent pneumonia for 2 years	Carcinoid bronchial adenoma	Right segmental bronchus	Bilobectomy		Free of recurrence for 9 years
13	11 years	f	Recurrent pneumonia for 3 months	Bronchial adenoma	Left main bronchus	Circumferential resection and left lower lobectomy		Free of recurrence for 20 years

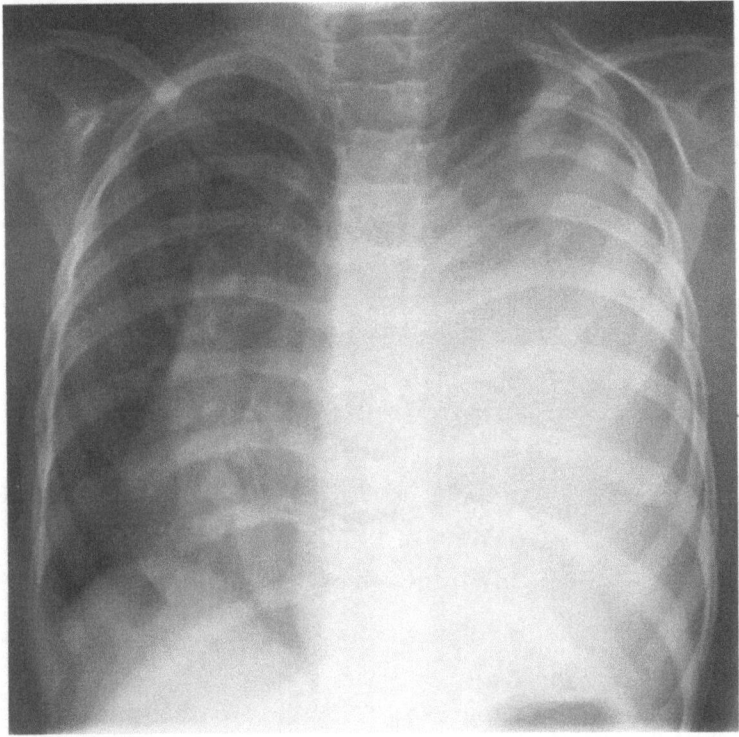

Fig. 1. A-P chest X-ray taken on 13 April 1978 in case 1 (date of birth 13 September 1973), showing pulmonary embryoma. Complete shadowing on left side and displacement of mediastinum to the right. Tracheobronchial tree not affected according to endoscopy

Chest X-ray: complete shadowing on the left side, with extensive mediastinal displacement to the right (Fig. 1). No evidence of bone or other metastases.

Treatment: Left-sided thoracotomy on 21 April 1978, revealing a crumbly tumour filling the whole of the pleural cavity. Almost complete excision of the tumour (tumour mass removed 1130 g).

Pathohistology: Pulmonary embryoma (Fig. 2a), ducts lined with cuboidal and or prismatic cylindrical epithelial cells, surrounded by mesenchymal parts. Figure 2b shows cartilaginous islands within very immature, highly polymorphic tumour tissue (recurrence).

Chemotherapy: Endoxan, Methotrexate, Fluorouracil, Velbe, Cosmegen, Oncovin, Adriamycin.

Radiotherapy for 5 weeks. Left basal recurrence 9 months thereafter (Fig. 3).

Further course: Second thoracotomy on 9 February 1979 and removal of two residual tumour nodes and a diaphragmatic metastasis.

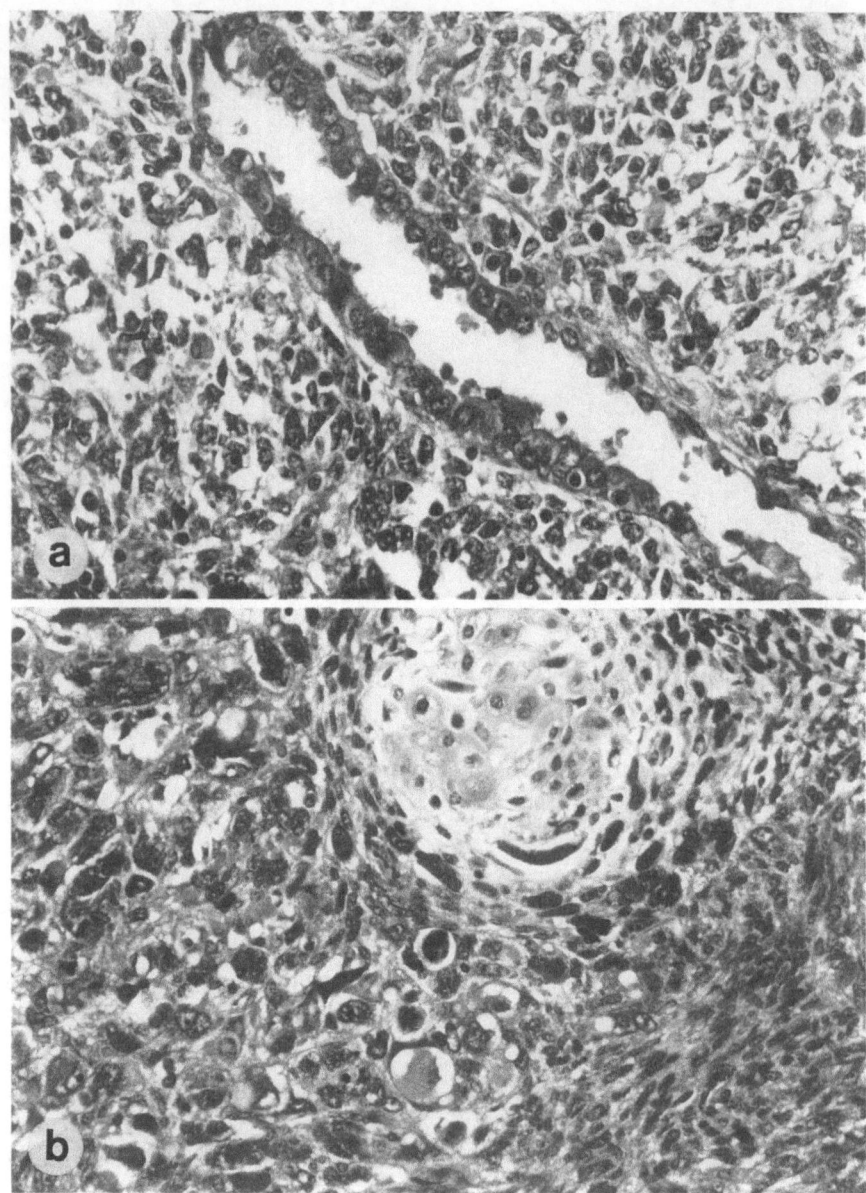

Fig. 2. a Primary tumour containing tubular structures lined with cuboidal epithelium, surrounded by a cellular stroma. **b** Recurrence with highly pleomorphic stroma containing giant cells and a few nodules of immature cartilage. H&E, ×110

Fig. 3. a Local recurrence (1 February 1979) at mid-base of left lung in case 1. At a second thoracotomy on 9 Feb 1979 the tumour was excised with partial resection of the diaphram. **b** Left lung free 10 days after second thoracotomy. Patient died 2 months later

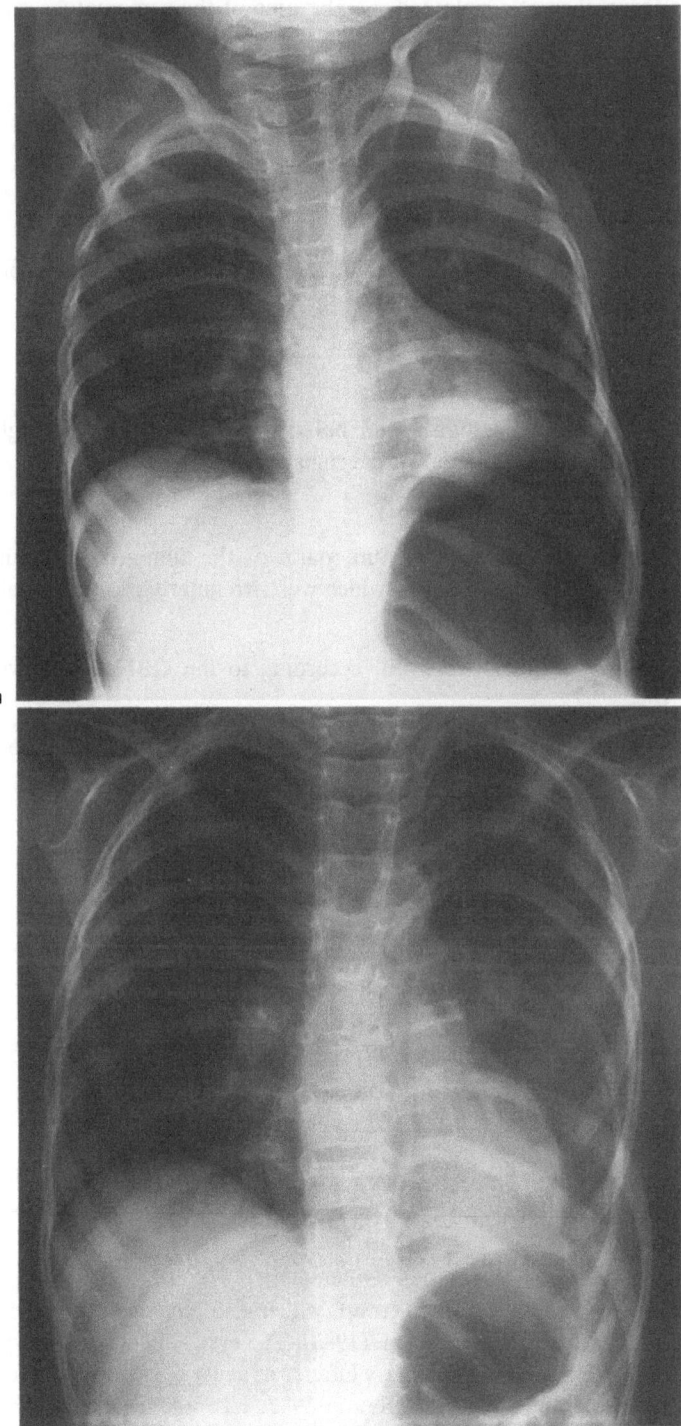

a

b
Fig. 3

Pathohistology: Recurrence of a pulmonary embryoma of the sarcomatous type (Fig. 2b).

Died on 20 April 1979, 1 year after first diagnosis.

Case 2

Boy, date of birth 21 May 1979

Anamnesis: Suspected lung cysts on the left side after chest X-ray for continuous coughing in this 3-year-old boy.

Thoracotomy (14 October 1980) and segmental resection S1 + S3 and resection of a cyst (S8).

Follow-up chest X-ray 2 years later showed polycyclic shadowing in the right lower lobe. Tentative diagnosis: tumour of the right lower lobe.

Treatment: Lobectomy (17 December 1982).

Pathohistology: Pulmonary blastoma: mature parts of the tumour containing fairly well-differentiated bronchial lumina, which were irregularly positioned and surrounded by undifferentiated matrix.

Chemotherapy: From 10 January 1983 on, according to the Ö81 rhabdomyosarcoma study.

Further course: CT scan revealed right parietal brain metastases (11 October 1983).

Died on 13 May 1984, at 17 months after first diagnosis.

Case 3

Date of birth 30 November 1965

Anamnesis: Coughing and weight loss over previous 6 weeks.

Chest X-ray: Shadowing in left lower lobe. Referral with diagnosis of pulmonary cyst in the left lower lobe.

Treatment: Thoracotomy and tumour enucleation on April 28, 1976.

Pathohistology: Malignant papillary pleural mesothelioma in the left lower lobe. Radiotherapy with ^{60}Co, 3000 cGy

Further course: Cured (findings of 1 January 1984).

Hamartomas of the lung are another group, which also includes the arteriovenous angiomas according to Ohtoma et al. (1983). The cystic adenomatoid type of this group may manifest itself even in early infancy as acute respiratory distress and lead to a life-threatening situation (Genton 1982; Izzo and Rickham 1968;

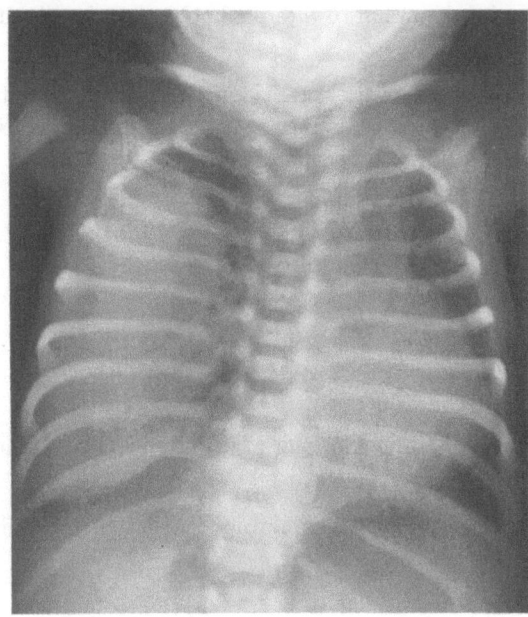

Fig. 4. Large tumour in right lung (case 7), with vesicular structures and gross mediastinal displacement to the right. Normal air distribution in the epigastrium

Taber and Schwarz 1972; Vos and Ekkelkamp 1979; Wolf et al. 1980). Examples of this were seen in cases 5 and 7 (Fig. 4).

We also found a malignant tumour in this group, a reticulosarcoma which had developed within a hamartoma (case 4).

Case 4

Date of birth 12 October 1976

Anamnesis: Chest X-ray for upper airways infection and immediate referral with suspected diagnosis of a right-sided pulmonary tumour.

Treatment: Segmental resection (S7) on 31 January 1978.

Pathohistology: Fibrous reticulosarcoma within a pulmonary hamartoma.

Chemotherapy: LSA_2L_2 protocol from 14 February 1978 onward.

Further course: 22 March 1979, local tumour recurrence with pleural effusion.

Died 14 months later.

Case 5

Date of birth 5 March 1964

Anamnesis: Cyanosis immediately after birth. Cardiac sounds displaced to the right.

Chest X-ray: shadowing of the left hemithorax with air bubbles. Referral with diagnosis of diaphragmatic hernia.

Treatment: Laparotomy on the first day of life, no evidence of a diaphragmatic hernia. Subsequent thoracotomy revealed a tumour $7 \times 5 \times 6$ cm in diameter in the left upper lobe and an atelectatic lower lobe.

Died on table following ligation of the upper lobe vessels.

Pathohistology: Hamartoma, similar to an alveolar dysplasia.

Case 6

Date of birth 12 April 1970

Anamnesis: Pneumonic episodes in the first trimester of life. Referral with diagnosis of pulmonary tumour.

Treatment: Thoracotomy (6th month) showed tumorous changes of the right upper and middle lobe, which were resected.

Pathohistology: Cystic hamartoma.

Case 9

Boy, date of birth 19 April 1977

Anamnesis: Hydrocephalus due to brain malformation (septum pellucidum cyst) required ventriculoperitoneal shunting in infancy. In addition the boy developed an increasing extracardiac right-left shunt and drumstick nails. Chest X-ray showed an arch-like shadow varying in density in the right lower lobe. Angiography revealed an extended arteriovenous angioma.

Treatment: at the age of 2 years 10 months clinical symptoms had completely disappeared, and the secondary changes receded following right lower lobectomy.

In the group of endobronchial tumours we found the so-called bronchial adenomas, two carcinoids and two mucoepidermoid tumours, located in the left main bronchus in two cases and in the right middle lobe and right middle bronchus in one case each. Circumferential resection, combined in one case with lower lobectomy, was carried out in two cases as an organ-preserving operation, and bilobectomy was performed in the other two cases. All these four children remain free of recurrence 5–20 years later; they are presented in detail in the next paper in this volume. In addition, we are able to include the patients seen at the paediatric University Hospital of Zurich (Stauffer 1982) and at the Paediatric University Hospital of Leipzig (Meissner et al. 1976). These include five more with malignant tumours (2 pulmonary blastomas, 2 sarcomas and 1 teratoma) and two more with bronchial adenomas (a carcinoid and a mucoepidermoid tumour of the left main bronchus) (Table 2 and 3).

Table 2. Lung tumours treated at the Paediatric Surgical Clinic Leipzig

Age	Sex	Anamnesis	Histology	Site	Treatment	Outcome
3 months	f	Abscess, pneumonia	CCAM, hamartoma	Right lower lobe	Bilob-ectomy	Well
4 months	m	Recurrent pneumonia	Hamartoma	Right middle lobe	Excision	Well
11 years	m	Incidental finding	Benign teratoma	Right middle lobe	Excision	Well
6 years	m	Pneumonia	Pulmonary blastoma	Right middle lobe	Segmental resection	Well for 4 years
3 years	f	Pneumonia	Pulmonary blastoma	Right middle lobe	Lob-ectomy	Died 4 months later
5.5 years	m	Thoracic wall tumour	Undiffer-entiated sarcoma	Right lung	Cyclo-phos-phamide + irra-diation	Death 8 months later

All were treated surgically. The bronchial adenomas seen at the Zurich Clinic were treated by bronchotomy and local tumour excision. In summary, there were 24 patients, among them 4 with pulmonary embryomas (mean age 5 years), 7 with hamartomas (mean age 2.6 years), 1 with hamartoma with malignant degeneration, 2 with arteriovenous aneurysms, 6 with bronchial adenomas (mean age 9 years), and 2 with teratomas, 1 of which was malignant. Pulmonary teratomas are also very rare (Gottschalk et al. 1980; Meissner et al. 1976).

A history of specific symptoms, such as cyanosis, right-left shunting and drumstick nails, was found only for children with arteriovenous aneurysms. All other children presented with unspecific signs of recurrent bronchial infections with pneumonia, particularly in bronchial adenomas, or the diagnosis was made incidentally (case 8).

Hamartomas led predominantly to respiratory distress in newborns. These cases can be compared with a group of seven cases in which differential diagnosis revealed that the pulmonary tumours present were benign processes (Table 4).

The patients with benign tumours had minor or major round shadows on X-ray. Two of the tumours were residual tuberculomas following antibiotically treated pneumonia, while the others were fluid-filled bronchial cysts. These cases have already been published elsewhere (Geissler et al. 1985/86).

Table 3. Lung tumours treated at the Paediatric Surgical Clinic of Zurich

Pat. no.	Age	Sex	Anamnesis	Histology	Site	Treatment	Outcome
1	12 years	f	Poly-cythaemia, embolism, drumstick fingers	A-V-aneurysm	Right lower lobe	Lob-ectomy	Well
2	2 years	f	Subfebrile tempera-ture	Histio-cytoma	Right upper lobe	Lob-ectomy	Well
3	8.5 years	m	Coughing, pneumonia	Bronchial adenoma, carcinoid	Left main bron-chus	Broncho-tomy, excision	Well
4	9.5 years	m	Recurrent pneumonia	Mucoepi-dermoid adenoma	Left main bron-chus	Broncho-tomy, excision	Well
5	3.5 years	f	Fever, pneumonia	Sarcoma	Total atel-ectasis, right lower + middle lobe	Pneumon-ectomy, resection of dia-phragm + peri-cardium	Death 3 months later
6	2.5 years	f	Coughing, fever, weight loss	Malignant teratoma, inter-mediate type	Left lower lobe	Lob-ectomy	Death 10 months later

Discussion

The absolute statutory requirement for notification of malignant diseases in the German Democratic Republic provides a good indication of the incidence of malignant lung tumours in childhood.

From 1952 to 1981 over 1.5 million new malignancies were diagnosed and registered. These included 10 800 cases in children below 15 years, accounting for 0.7% of the cases registered.

In the 10-year period from 1968 to 1977 only 8 malignant tumours of lung, trachea and bronchi were found among 4092 children with malignant diseases, 1 in an infant under 1 year of age; 1 in the age group 1–5 years; 1 in the 6- to 10-year

Table 4. Benign entities in the differential diagnosis of lung tumours

Pat. no.	Age	Sex	Anamnesis	Histology	Site	Treatment	Outcome
1	12 years	f	Left-sided pneumonia for 2 years	Tuber-culoma	Left lower lobe	Excision	Free of recurrence for 6 years
2	6 years	m	Pneumonia	Tuber-culoma	Right upper	Segmental resection	Free of recurrence for 7 years
3	11 years	f	Incidental finding	Broncho-genic cyst	Left lower lobe	Excision	Free of recurrence for 10 years
4	1 year	f	Bronchitis	Broncho-genic cyst	Right lower lobe	Excision	Free of recurrence for 6 years
5	11 years	f	Incidental finding	Bronchi-ectasis, cyst	Right lower lobe	Excision + bron-chus re-section	Free of recurrence for 5 years
6	3 years	f	Bronchitis	Bronchial cyst	Tra-chea[a]	Excision + slitting	Recur-rence
7	5 months	m	Incidental finding	Extra-lobar se-questration	Media-stinum[a]	Excision	Free of recurrence

[a] Radiologically located in the lung.

group; and 5 in the 11- to 15-year group. Thus, only 0.2% of the 4092 children with malignancies had malignant tumours of trachea, bronchi and lungs.

Similar findings were reported by Marsden and Scholtz (1976), who in a total of 1.5 million registered malignancies observed only 2207 malignant tumours in children up to 1976, and among these only 4 malignant lung tumours (1 squamous epithelial carcinoma, 1 malignant teratoma, 1 undifferentiated carcinoma and 1 pulmonary blastoma). Whereas bronchial carcinoma is one of the most common malignancies in adults, only about 30 cases of pulmonary blastoma in adults have been published (Karzioglu and Someren 1974; Kennedy and Prior 1976; Marsden and Scholtz 1976; Ohtoma et al. 1983; Weinblatt et al. 1982). In contrast, in our material at least, pulmonary blastoma was the most frequent malignant lung tumour in childhood, followed by the various forms of semimalignant to malignant bronchial adenomas, which are in turn also rare tumours in adults (Andrassy et al. 1977; Keller and Helwig 1981; Metze et al. 1981; Stauffer 1982; Wurnig 1978).

Using the classification of lung tumours of the Austrian Society of Pathology (Gibbons et al. 1981), among the 11 different groups in group I (epithelial tu-

Table 5. Primary lung tumours in childhood (Jones et al. 1976, modified by Stauffer 1982)

Benign	Malignant
Hamartomas	Bronchial adenomas
Papillomas or papillomatosis	Bronchial carcinomas
Histiocytomas	Sarcomas of trachea, bronchi and lungs
Differentiated (so-called adult) teratomas	Pulmonary blastomas
	Undifferentiated (embryonic) teratomas

Table 6. Classification of lung tumours in childhood (Meissner et al. 1976)

I. Embryonic tumors

1. Pulmonary blastomas
2. Hamartomas
   a. Localized hamartoma
   b. Diffuse hamartoma
   c. Cystic hamartoma
   d. Fibroleiomyomatous hamartoma
3. Teratomas

II. Mesenchymal tumours

1. Benign tumours
2. Sarcomas

III. Epithelial tumours

1. Bronchial adenomas
2. Bronchial carcinoids   80% [a]
3. Cylindromas   5%–10% [a]
4. Mucoepidermoid tumours   2%– 3% [a]
5. Bronchial carcinomas

[a] According to Keller and Helwig 1981.

mours) we found only the various forms of bronchial adenomas, and not carcinoma, in group VII four pulmonary blastomas and 2 teratomas, and in group XI seven hamartomas, one with malignant degeneration. We conclude therefore that a classification of lung tumours in childhood according to an adult scheme is unfavourable and prefer the classification according to Jones and Campbell (1976) (modified by Stauffer 1982; Table 5) or to Meissner et al. (1976) (Table 6).

The pulmonary blastoma or pulmonary embryoma according to Barnard (1952) and Spencer (1961) is the typical lung tumour in childhood. Similar to 'nephroblastoma', the term pulmonary blastoma was chosen because these tumours obviously originate from the primitive pluripotential mesenchyma of the pulmonary blastoma. Since 1977, about 38 cases have been described in the literature (Fung et al. 1977; Karzioglu and Someren 1974; Kennedy and Prior 1976), 30 in male and 8 in female patients, their ages ranging from 2 months to 77 years with an average of 39 years. Of these patients, 19 died within 2 years after diagnosis and 19 survived for more than 2 years. The relatively late onset of an embryonal tumour can be explained by the fact that lung tissue matures for at least 10 years after birth, in contrast to other organs where maturation is completed much earlier (Spencer 1961). Fung et al. (1977) and McCann et al. (1976) emphasize that, in contrast to bronchial carcinoma and carcinosarcoma of the lung, pulmonary blastoma grows more peripherally rather than endobronchially. The pulmonary blastoma is composed of two different primitive cell types, which may differentiate into bronchial cells and chondrocytes. Biological behaviour is therefore unpredictable (McCann et al. 1976). Karzioglu and Someren (1974) found very different courses in 22 cases: relatively benign forms with long-term survival, but also malignant forms with local recurrences and metastases. They were not able to find reliable histological criteria for prognosis. The characteristic pathohistological changes are shown in Fig. 2. The tumour seems to respond to chemotherapy following surgery, but relapses frequently, then showing a more malignant behaviour (Fig. 2b). There was slow growth also in our own case, which corresponds to reports in the literature (Fung et al. 1977; Karzioglu and Someren 1974) where the patients often survived longer than 1 year after diagnosis. The extrabronchial growth rarely allows diagnosis by endoscopy or cytology. A lack of experience with optimal chemotherapy might be the reason for the poor results.

Weinblatt et al. (1982) described an accumulation of pulmonary blastomas in six cases of cystic lung disease. Hence, patients with cystic lung disease should be carefully followed up. Our material, also included a patient with cystic lung disease who later developed pulmonary blastoma (case 2).

Endobronchial tumours (adenomas, cylindromas, mucoepidermoid tumours) are another group, generating a lot of interest, particularly as far as therapy is concerned (Andrassy et al. 1977; Keller and Helwig 1981; Metze et al. 1981). They will be described in detail in the next chapter. Here it is merely remarked that endoscopy is the most important diagnostic method, yielding correct diagnosis in nearly 100%. If endoscopy was performed in recurrent pneumonias in good time, these cases were diagnosed more properly. Endoscopic resection formerly in use was abandoned because of the high recurrence rate, the danger of massive intraoperative bleeding and the possibility of malignant degeneration years later (Andrassy et al. 1977; Wurnig 1967).

The therapy of choice is either circumferential resection (Wurnig 1967, 1968) with or without additional lobectomy or, if possible, local excision of the tumour via bronchotomy (Stauffer 1982). Circumferential resection, which is technically more sophisticated, seems to be safer in the sense of more radical. According to more recent reports, mere circumferential resection seems to be possible in the presence of even severe changes peripheral to the tumour, since intensive aftercare enables recovery of the peripheral damaged lung tissue.

Table 7. Diagnostic procedures for suspected lung tumours in children

Procedures	Indispensable/ optional	Step
Lateral and A-P chest X-ray	Indispensable	1
Tomography	Indispensable	2
CT scan	Indispensable	2
Bronchoscopy	Indispensable	1
Bronchography	Indispensable	2
Inhalation scintiscan	Optional	3
Perfusion scintiscan	Optional	3
Exclusion of tuberculosis	Indispensable	1
Exclusion of mycosis	Indispensable	1
Ultrasound	Indispensable	1

In their cystic form, lung hamartomas, recently termed congenital adenomatoid malformation of the lungs, are frequently life-threatening even in the neonatal period (Genton 1982; Izzo and Rickham 1968; Stauffer 1982; Taber and Schwarz 1972; Vos and Ekkelkamp 1979; Wolf et al. 1980).

Others present on X-ray predominantly as solid shadows and harmless small round foci (case 8), which may, however, also lead to life-threatening situations in the neonatal period because of their considerable size. These tumours may then be considered air-filled lung tumours (Fig. 4). It is important to point out that one of our cases (case 4) developed malignant degeneration (see also Weinblatt et al. 1982). The cystic forms already causing symptoms in the neonatal period must be differentiated from diaphragmatic hernias, particularly by paediatricians who use the abdominal approach for diaphragmatic hernia. In contrast to diaphragmatic hernia, cystic lung hamartomas cause abdominal distention, and plain abdominal X-rays show air-filled bowel slings in the abdomen. Cases of this type have frequently been described (Wolf et al. 1980). Following correct preoperative diagnosis a thoracic approach (thoracotomy) will be chosen, reducing the perioperative risk considerably (case 5).

Since lung tumours are so rare in childhood, there may be little experience available, leading to uncertainty in the individual case as far as diagnosis and therapy are concerned. (Table 7). Anamnesis and clinical symptoms correspond to unspecific recurrent bronchial infections whose site and extension are revealed by chest X-rays. The suspicion of a tumour really arises only if the pathological changes are resistant to antibiotic therapy, recover incompletely, or recur. According to Stauffer (1982), this may cause considerable delay before proper treatment can be started. Among other diagnostic methods, bronchoscopy is the adequate procedure for endobronchial tumours (adenomas). Biopsy allows correct diagnosis and further therapy. Exploratory thoracotomy may not be helpful in every case of extrabronchially growing tumours or unclear findings, since lung tumours are seldom superficially located and may be missed in the early stages if biopsy is attempted.

Summary

From the patient material of three paediatric surgical centres and the patient material of the paediatric surgical hospitals of Zurich, Switzerland and Leipzig, GDR, 24 cases of lung and bronchial tumours are reported. The aim of this review is to show a spectrum of the cases observed in our region. The most frequent of these very rare tumours was pulmonary blastoma, followed by endobronchial adenoma in its different variants. Since only the latter can be endoscopically diagnosed, endoscopy should be carried out as early as possible when the diagnosis is not clear. Cystic lung disease seems to be particularly frequently associated with pulmonary blastomas. Uncertainties in diagnosis and therapy owing to the rareness of these diseases cause further problems.

Résumé

Observation de 24 patients présentant des tumeurs pulmonaires et bronchiques traités dans trois centres de chirurgie infantile et dans les cliniques de chirurgie infantile de Leipzig et de Zurich. Il s'agissait avant tout de donner une vue d'ensemble des cas observés dans notre région. La forme la plus fréquente parmi ces tumeurs extrêmement rares, est ici le blastome pulmonaire, vient ensuite l'adénome endobronchial et ses variantes. Puisque seul ce dernier peut être diagnostiqué par endoscopie, il convient de pratiquer une endoscopie le plus tôt possible dans les cas doutex. Il semble que les kystes aériens du poumon soient très souvent associés au blastome pulmonaire. L'incertitude règne souvent dans le domaine du diagnostic et de la thérapeutique car ces affections sont extrêmement rares, ce qui n'est pas sans poser des problèmes supplémentaires.

Zusammenfassung

Es wird über 24 Fälle von Lungen- und Bronchialtumoren berichtet, die aus dem gesamten Krankengut dreier kinderchirurgischer Zentren unter Einbeziehung der Kinderchirurgischen Kliniken Leipzig und Zürich gesammelt wurden. Zweck dieser Darstellung war es, ein Spektrum der beobachteten Fälle in unserer Region aufzuzeigen. Die häufigste Form dieser sehr seltenen Tumoren war das pulmonale Blastom, gefolgt vom endobronchialen Adenom in seinen verschiedenen Varianten. Der endoskopischen Diagnostik ist nur das letztere zugänglich, daher sollte bei unklaren Prozessen schon möglichst frühzeitig die endoskopische Diagnostik durchgeführt werden. Zystische Lungenerkrankungen scheinen gehäuft mit pulmonalen Blastomen einherzugehen. Die Seltenheit dieser Erkrankungen bringt aufgrund der Unsicherheit in diagnostischer und therapeutischer Hinsicht weitere Probleme.

References

Andrassy RJ, Feldtman RW, Stanford W (1977) Bronchial carcinoid tumors in children and adolescents. J Pediatr Surg 12:513–517

Barnard WG (1952) Embryoma of the lung. Thorax 7:299

Breitenecker G, Budka H, Denk H, Feigl W, Hanak H, Holzner JH, Kessler J, Köhler H, Lederer B, Leibl B, Obiditsch-Mayer I, Wuketich S (1968) Histologische Tumorklassifikation. Histopathologische Nomenklatur und Klassifikation der Tumoren und tumorartigen Veränderungen. Springer, Vienna New York

Fung CH, Lo JW, Yonan TN, et al (1977) Pulmonary blastoma, an ultrastructural study with a brief review of literature and discussion of pathogenesis. Cancer 39:153–163

Geißler W, Wurnig P, Klos I (1985/86) Formen und Bedeutung von Trachealstenosen. Padiatr Prax 32:487–503

Genton N (1982) Kongenitale Lungencysten. In: Bettex M, Genton N, Stockmann M (eds) Kinderchirurgie: Diagnostik, Indikation, Therapie und Prognose, 2nd edn, vol 5. Thieme, Stuttgart, p 173

Gibbons JRP, Mckeown F, Field TW (1981) Pulmonary blastoma with hilar lymphnode metastases. Cancer 47:152–155

Gottschalk E, Lichey C, Friedrich U (1980) Thorakale Teratome bei Kindern. Z Kinderchir 29:303–312

Izzo C, Rickham PP (1968) Neonatal pulmonary hamartoma. J Pediatr Surg 3:77

Jones PG, Campbell PE (1976) Tumours of infancy and childhood. Blackwell, Oxford

Karzioglu ZA, Someren AO (1974) Pulmonary blastoma, a case report and review of the literature. Am J Chir Pathol 61:287–295

Keller KM, Helwig H (1981) Bronchialcarcinoide im Kindesalter – Fallbericht und Übersicht. Klin Padiatr 193:355–361

Kennedy A, Prior AL (1976) Pulmonary blastoma, the report of two cases and a review of the literature. Thorax 31:776

Marsden HB, Scholtz CL (1976) Pulmonary blastoma. Virchows Arch [A] 372:161–165

McCann MP, Yoo Shi Fu, Kay S (1976) Pulmonary blastoma, a light and electron microscopic study. Cancer 38:789–797

Meissner F, Hofmann V, Willnow U (1976) Primäre Lungentumoren im Säuglings- und Kindesalter. Z Kinderchir 18:117–132

Metze H, Fenne D, Caesar R (1981) Mucoepidermoider Bronchialdrüsentumor im Kindesalter. Chir Prax 28:691–695

Ohtoma K, Araki T, Yashiro N, Ilio M (1983) Pulmonary blastoma in children. Radiology 147:101–104

Spencer H (1961) Pulmonary blastoma. J Pathol Bacteriol 82:161–165

Stauffer UG (1982) Lungentumoren und Lungenmetastasen. In: Betex M, Genton N, Stockmann M (eds) Kinderchirurgie, Diagnostik, Indikation, Therapie und Prognose, 2nd edn, vol 5. Thieme, Stuttgart, p 218

Taber P, Schwarz DE (1972) Cystic lung lesion in a newborn: Congenital cystic adenomatoid malformation of the lung. J Pediatr Surg 7:366

Vos A, Ekkelkamp S (1979) Congenital cystic adenomatoid malformation of the lung in newborn. Z Kinderchir 27:125–129

Weinblatt ME, Siegel SE, Isaacs H (1982) Pulmonary blastoma associated with cystic lung disease. Cancer 49:669–671

Willnow U, Hofmann V (1974) Zur Morphologie und Histogenese der primären Lungentumoren des Kindes. Helv Paediatr Acta 29:425–438

Wolf SA, Hertzler JH, Philipat AE (1980) Cystic adenomatoid dysplasia of the lung. J Pediatr Surg 15:925

Wurnig P (1967) Technische Vorteile bei der Hauptbronchusresektion rechts und links. Thorax-chir Vask Chir 15:16

Wurnig P (1968) Ein Fall von Hauptbronchusresektion bei einem 11jährigen Mädchen. Z Kinderchir 5:343

Wurnig P (1971) Der kindliche Thoraxtumor. Langenbecks Arch f Chirurgie, Band 329, S 123–125, 329:123 (Kongreßbericht)

Wurnig P (1978) Maligne Tumoren im Kindesalter. Chirurgie der Gegenwart, vol VII K 19. Urban and Schwarzenberg, Munich

Endotracheal and Endobronchial Tumours in Childhood

N. Augustin[1], S. Hofmann-v. Kap-Herr[2], and P. Wurnig[2]

Introduction

The frequency of bronchial adenomas is reported in the literature as 1%–10% of all resected lung tumours in all age groups (Andrassy et al. 1977; Bean and Haldenby 1976; Lack et al. 1983). In childhood they are the second most frequent type of lung tumour. The following types are differentiated according to pathohistological findings: carcinoids (80%–90%), cylindromas (12%–15%), and mucoepidermoid tumours (2%–3%) (Batson et al. 1966). About three-quarters of bronchial adenomas are localised in the main and lobar bronchi. They must be considered potentially malignant, since metastases occur in 5%–20% of cases (Condon and Philipp 1962; Wellons et al. 1976).

Since 1962, 41 case reports of bronchial adenomas in childhood have been published (Ali Madani 1977; Bean and Haldenby 1976; Bharani et al. 1976; Breyer et al. 1980; Condon and Philipp 1962; Conlan et al. 1978; Debus et al. 1971; Deparedes et al. 1970; Gandjour and Stapenhorst 1972; Logan et al. 1970; McCarthy and Gallus 1979; McDougall et al. 1980; Mullins and Barnes 1979; Nakagawara et al. 1979; Nunez et al. 1966; Panabokke et al. 1971; Verska and Connolly 1968; Wellons et al. 1976; Wurnig 1968). Metastases were already present in 4 cases. One striking feature was that mucoepidermoid tumours, only of minor interest in the series published so far, accounted for nearly 50% (17 cases) (Batson et al. 1966). Mucoepidermoid tumours are obviously of a similar significance to carcinoids in childhood.

Patients

Two patients with bronchial tumours have been operated on in the Department of Paediatric Surgery of the Mautner Markhof Children's Hospital in Vienna and two in the Paediatric Surgical University Hospital of Mainz since 1965 (Table 1).

The children presented with symptoms of chronically recurrent bronchial infections over several months to some years. In three cases foreign body aspiration was suspected. Medical examination necessitated bronchoscopy in all four patients, which allowed the correct diagnosis. Treatment took the form of pneumon-

[1]Paediatric Surgical Hospital, D-6500 Mainz, FRG.
[2]Department of Paediatric Surgery, Mautner Markhof Children's Hospital of Vienna, A-1030 Vienna III, Austria.

Table 1. Endotracheal tumours in children reported

Pat. no.	Age	Sex	Symptoms	Tumour	Locali- zation	Treat- ment	Follow-up
1	12 years	f	Cough and recurrent pneumonia for 1 year	Mucoepi- dermoid tumour	Right middle lobe	Bilob- ectomy	Free of recurrence for 5 years
2	8 years	m	Recurrent pneumonia	Malignant mucoepi- dermoid tumour	Left main bron- chus	Circum- ferential resection	Free of recurrence for 6 years
3	8 years	f	Recurrent pneumonia for 2 years	Carcinoid (bronchial adenoma)	Right middle bron- chus	Bilob- ectomy	Free of recurrence for 9 years
4	11 years	f	Recurrent pneumonia for 3 months	Bronchial adenoma	Left main bron- chus	Circum- ferential resection and lower lobectomy	Free of recurrence for 20 years

ectomy in one case, bilobectomy in one, and circumferential resection in two cases, combined with lobectomy in one of these (Wurnig 1968).

Case Reports

Case 1

An 8-year-old boy was admitted to hospital in January 1975 for chronic bronchitis and recurrent pulmonary infections. The first coughing attacks had been noted in 1970, with left chest pain at rest and during activity. Herpes zoster infection of the left costal arch had occurred 6 months later.

Clinical findings: The general and nutritional state was reduced and breathing sounds over the left lung diminished. Increased blood sedimentation rate, slight leucocytosis, and moderate anaemia were also observed.

Pulmonary function test: A restrictive and obstructive ventilatory disturbance was revealed.

Chest X-ray: Mediastinal displacement to the left was seen (Fig. 1a).

Bronchoscopy: An obstructive tumour in the left main bronchus was seen.

Biopsy: The tumour proved to be a bronchial adenoma without evidence of malignancy.

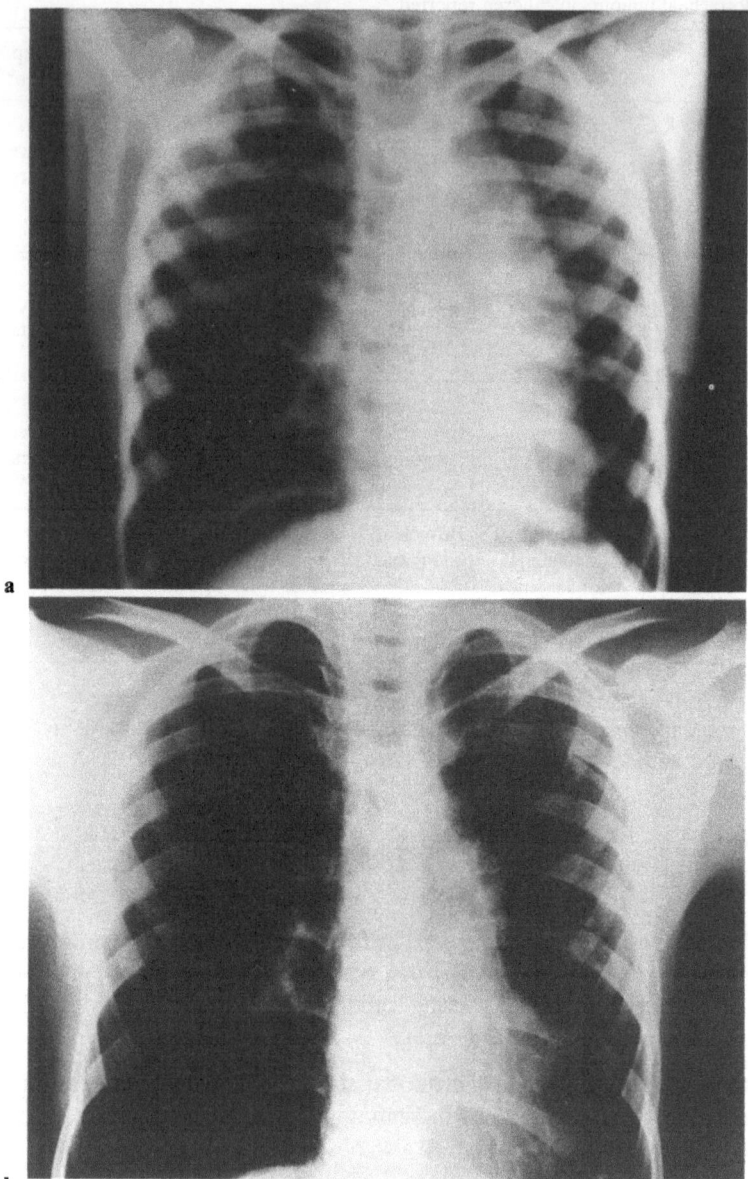

Fig. 1a–d. Case 1: **a** Preoperative chest X-ray, showing slight mediastinal displacement to the left. **b** Chest X-ray 6 years postoperatively, showing persisting minimal mediastinal displacement following circumferential resection. **c** Bronchogram: large filling defect in the left main bronchus *(arrows).* **d** Intraoperative view: infiltration of the left main bronchus caused by the endobronchial tumour clearly visible

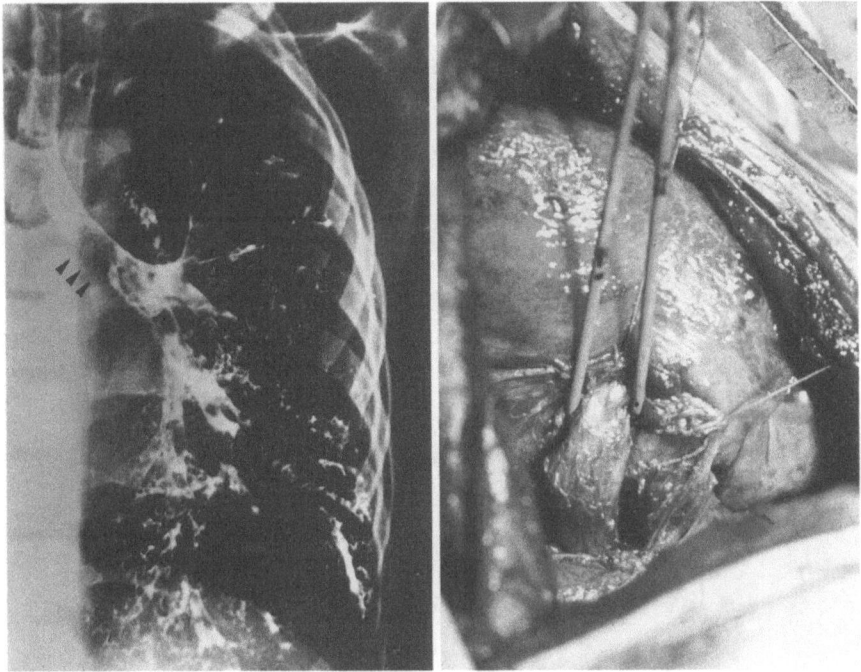

c   d

Fig. 1c–d

Bronchography: A defect in the left main bronchus was seen, obstructing nearly the whole lumen over 1.5 cm (Fig. 1c).

Surgical treatment: Thoracotomy via the left 4th intercostal space revealed an extensively collapsed, nearly hepatized left lung with extensive atelectatic and pneumonic changes, mainly in the lower lobe. Subsequent preparation and exposure of the left main bronchus disclosed thickening of the bronchial wall about 1.5 cm below the carina. On the basis of these findings, pneumonectomy and circumferential bronchial resection with or without resection of the lower lobe were considered for treatment. The latter procedure was selected, to avoid restriction of lung function later on.

Pathohistological findings: In contrast to the biopsy result, a malignant mucoepidermoid tumour was recognized.

Postoperative course: Development took a normal course.

Follow-up chest X-ray after 6 years: No substantial pathological findings were revealed (Fig. 1b).

Case 2

A 8-year-old girl was admitted to hospital on 2 February 1965 for recurrent pneumonia after the diagnosis of a benign tumour in the left main bronchus

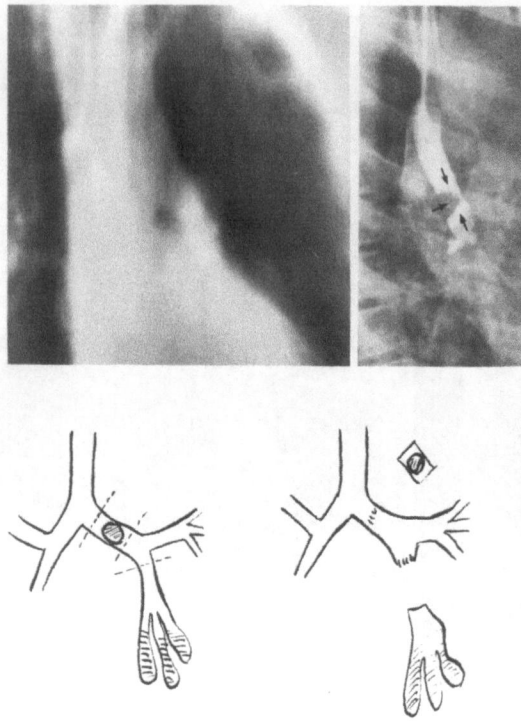

Fig. 2. Case 2: *Left*, tomogram; *right*, bronchogram; tumour in the left main bronchus easily recognizable

Fig. 3. Schematic of operative procedure applied in case 2: *left*, preoperative state; *right*, resection and anastomosis

(Fig. 2). Extensive bronchiectasis was already present in the atelectatic left lower lobe. Endoscopy and CT scan revealed a benign, bean-sized tumour immediately below the carina, obstructing the left main bronchus entirely.

We decided against endoscopic biopsy because of the narrowness of the bronchial tree (5 mm), and as benign tumours in particular sometimes give rise to massive bleeding. On 15 February 1965 we performed resection of the tumour-bearing part of the left main bronchus with subsequent bronchial anastomosis and lower lobectomy (surgeon PW) (Fig. 3). The postoperative course was entirely uneventful and the patient is free of symptoms 20 years later.

The clinical, radiological and bronchoscopic follow-up examinations of the remaining two patients have not revealed any evidence of recurrence or metastases up to the present day.

Discussion

Chronically recurrent bronchial infections in bronchial adenoma caused by tumour obstruction may frequently be evident over quite long periods. The most frequent radiological findings are pneumonia and atelectasis due to obstruction. Bronchoscopy is the most effective diagnostic measure, enabling localization and biopsy of bronchial adenomas in 80%–90% of cases (Bean and Haldenby 1976). Care must be taken at biopsy since the tumours are normally well vascularized and there is often bleeding subsequently (Wilkins et al. 1963). Exact pathohistological differentiation is not always possible by means of biopsy. Thus, among 9 biopsies in the 17 mucoepidermoid tumours mentioned above, 5 led to faulty diagnoses. Bronchography or tomography usually show the defects caused by the tumour, sometimes complete bronchial obstruction and possibly secondary bronchiectasis.

The following possibilities must be considered in differential diagnosis: foreign-body aspiration, bronchial asthma, pneumonia, tuberculosis and other granulomatous infections, and cystic fibrosis of the pancreas with secondary bronchiectases. The immotile cilia syndrome must now also be borne in mind and excluded.

The treatment of bronchial adenomas depends on tumour localization and extension, the presence or absence of metastases and the extent of secondary changes. The treatment is basically surgical, since endoscopic resection does not guarantee radical excision (Wurnig 1967), in addition to which extrabronchial parts of cylindromas may be missed. This procedure is therefore now omitted. Moreover, endoscopical resection was of only limited applicability in children, because of the narrow bronchial tree (Wilkins et al. 1963; Wurnig 1968).

The chance of organ-preserving operative procedures is greater with earlier diagnosis of the tumours. These procedures must be attempted with regard to avoiding long-term damage, which is particularly unfavourable in childhood, when centrally localized tumours without metastases are concernced.

Besides bronchotomy with tumour excision in the case of pediculated polyps, bronchial resections (sleeve resection, circumferential resection) come into are the main procedures to consider.

Most papers describing bronchial resection for bronchial adenomas report uneventful postoperative courses with no evidence of recurrences during follow-up periods of 1–20 years (case 2).

Moreover, bronchial resection is applied for the correction of cicatricial changes following bronchial rupture in children and, more rarely, in the treatment of tuberculous bronchial stenoses (Wurnig 1968).

Our experience indicates that circumferential resections provide good long-term results.

Some technical manoeuvers, however, must be taken into account in circumferential resection in childhood. Preparation should provide for extended mobilization of the lung, as for pneumonectomy. The central parts of the tumorous bronchus must be precisely exposed, and in particular the bronchial artery should be ligated prior to opening of the bronchus to prevent haemorrhage while the bronchus is open. Ventilation of the other lung parts without detriment to the procedure must also be ensured prior to opening of the bronchus, which necessitates bronchial blockage by means of a proper tube. This, however, may be difficult in the small bronchial systems of children. In these cases atraumatic, temporary clamping of the bronchus has proved useful, being easily performed with no

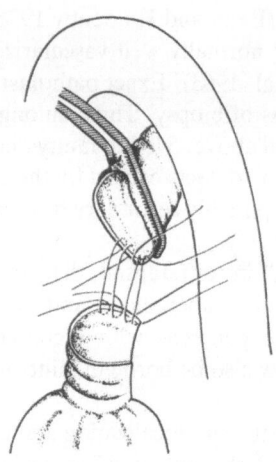

Fig. 4. Operative technique for main bronchus resection and atraumatic clamping of the left main bronchus. Prepared medial sutures, led from the exterior to the interior and vice versa and tied outside. The atraumatic clamp makes it possible to pull the bronchus out below the aorta. (From Wurnig 1967 by permission)

damage to the bronchial system and allowing the surgeon to operate undisturbed while the remaining lung is normally ventilated. Today we perform bronchial anastomosis with absorbable suture material and the sutures are tied outside to prevent irritation of the lumen (Fig. 4). It must be decided individually in each case whether an additional lobectomy may be required. Preservation of the upper lobe can even be possible, and the tumour is localized in the main bronchus, necessitating lower lobectomy, as is shown in the technique used in case 2 (Fig. 3). Nowadays the options of antibiotic therapy and inhalation treatment may improve even massive changes in the lung that have already been present for quite a long time, as could be shown in several cases of traumatic main bronchus stenosis successfully repaired after some months.

Summary

Following a review of the literature on the most common types of endobronchial tumours (carcinoid cylindromas and mucoepidermoid tumours), four cases of such bronchial tumours in children are reported. Two of them underwent isolated bronchial resection, whereas one of the others had to undergo bilobectomy in addition and the other, pneumonectomy. The patients remained free of recurrences after a follow-up of 5–20 years. The advantage of circumferential resection and some technical aspects are discussed.

Résumé

Après avoir passé en revue la littérature consacrée aux formes les plus courantes de tumeurs endobronchiques (cylindromes carcinoïdes et tumeurs muco-épidermoides) les auteurs traitent de quatre cas d'enfants présentant ces tumeurs. Deux d'entre eux subirent une résection bronchique uniquement, les deux autres eurent à subir également une bilobectomie et une pneumonectomie respectivement. Les patients ont été suivis de cinq à vingt ans et il n'y a pas eu de récidive. Il est question aussi des avantages présentés par la technique de résection décrite.

Zusammenfassung

Nach einer Literaturzusammenstellung über die häufigsten Typen der endobronchialen Tumoren (Karzinoide Zylindrome und Mukoepidermoidtumoren) wird über 4 Fälle solcher Bronchialtumoren bei Kindern berichtet. Zwei davon wurden einer isolierten Bronchusresektion unterzogen, bei zweien mußte gleichzeitig entweder eine Bilobektomie oder eine Pneumonektomie vorgenommen werden. Die Fälle sind zwischen 5 und 20 Jahren rezidivfrei geheilt. Die Vorteile der Manschettenresektion werden mit einigen technischen Bemerkungen dargestellt.

References

Ali Madani MA (1977) Mucoepidermoid-bronchial adenoma with unusual pattern of growth. NY State J Med 77:1283–1285

Andrassy RJ, Feldtmann RW, Stanford W (1977) Bronchial carcinoid tumors in children and adolescents. J Pediatr Surg 12/4:513–517

Batson JF, Gale JW, Hickey RC (1966) Bronchial adenomata. Arch Surg 92:623–630

Bean DM, Haldenby DA (1976) Endobronchial adenomata in children. J Otolaryngol 5/6:519–522

Bharani SN, Arbeit JM, Hyde JS, Dainauskas JR, Wilson RR (1976) Mucoepidermoid tumor of trachea. Chest 70/6:782–784

Breyer RH, Dainauskas JR, Jensik RJ, Faber LP (1980) Mucoepidermoid carcinoma of the trachea and bronchus. The case for conservative resection. Ann Thorac Surg 29:197–204

Condon VR, Philipp EW (1962) Bronchial adenoma in children: a review of the literature and report of three cases. Ann J Roentgenol 88:543–554

Conlan AA, Payne WS, Woolner LB, Sanderson DR (1978) Adenoid cystic carcinoma (cylindroma) and mucoepidermoid carcinoma of the bronchus. Affection survival. J Thorac Cardiovasc Surg 76:369–377

Debus PJ, Lewis MJ, Shepherd DJ (1971) Mucoepidermoid tumor of the bronchus in a child. Br J Dis Chest 65:130–133

Deparedes CG, Pierce WS, Groff DB, Waldhausen JA (1970) Bronchogenic tumors in children. Arch Surg 100:574–576

Gandjour A, Stapenhorst K (1972) Angeborene Lungenfehlbildungen als Notfälle im Säuglingsalter. Monatschr Kinderheilkd 120:57–61

Lack EE, Harris GBC, Eraklis AJ, Vawter GF (1983) Primary bronchial tumors in childhood. Cancer 51:492–497

Liebow AA (1952) Tumors of the lower respiratory tract. In: Subcommittee on Oncology of the Committee on Pathology of the National Research Council (eds) Atlas of tumor pathology, sect 5. Armed Forces Institute of Pathology, Washington, p 45

Logan WDJR, Sehdeva J, Hatcher CR, Abbott OA (1970) Tracheobronchial adenomas. Am Surg 36:359–364

McCarthy DJ, Gallus J (1979) Bronchial adenoma in a child. Report of a case. Rocky Mt Med J 76:83–84

McDougall JC, Unni K, Corenstein A, Connel EJ (1980) Carcinoid and mucoepidermoid carcinoma of bronchus in children. Ann Otol Rhinol Laryngol 89:425–427

Mullins JD, Barnes RP (1979) Childhood bronchial mucoepidermoid tumors. A case report and review of the literature. Cancer 44:315–322

Nakagawara A, Keda K, Ohgami H (1979) Mucoepidermoid tumor of the bronchus in an infant. J Pediatr Surg 14:608–609

Nunez VA, Spjut HJ, Rosenber HS (1966) Bronchial adenomas in children. Tex Med 61:683–686

Panabokke RG, Stephen SJ, Bragoda CG (1971) Incidence of bronchial adenoma in Ceylon, with case report on a child. Ceylon Med J 15:110–113

Verska JJ, Connolly JE (1968) Bronchial adenomas in children. J Thorac Cardiovasc Surg 55:411–417

Wellons HA Jr, Eggleston P, Golden GT, Allen MS (1976) Bronchial adenoma in childhood. Two case reports and review of literature. Am J Dis Child 130:301–304

Wilkins EW Jr, Darting RC, Soutter L, Sniffen RC (1963) A continuing clinical survey of adenomas of the trachea and bronchus in a general hospital. J Thorac Cardiovasc Surg 46:279

Wurnig P (1967) Technische Vorteile bei der Hauptbronchusresektion rechts und links. Thoraxchirurgie – vaskuläre Chirurgie 15:16–25

Wurnig P (1968) Ein Fall von linksseitiger Hauptbronchusresektion bei einem elfjährigen Mädchen. Z Kinderchir 5/3:343–349

Subject Index

Progress in Pediatric Surgery

Volume 19

Long-gap Esophageal Atresia
Prenatal Diagnosis of
Congenital Malformations

Editor: P. Wurnig

1986. 86 figures. XII, 205 pages. ISBN 3-540-15881-2

The goal of this series is to publish the latest information dealing with pathophysiology, diagnosis, therapy, and post-operative treatment in the field of pediatric surgery.

This is the second volume to be published by Springer-Verlag. The first part focuses on the problems of long-gap esophageal atresia where the authors evaluate newer procedures against the original methods of treatment. The section includes such topics as: current surgical strategies with regard to endoscopy anastomosis, colonic interposition, esophageal replacement, gastric tube esophagoplasty, tracheal stenosis, end-to-end anastomosis under maximal tension, Rehbein's olive technique, gastroesophageal reflux following repair of esophageal atresia, pressure-induced growth, and dacron-patch, aortopexy. The second section then discusses the significance and consequences of prenatal diagnosis of congenital malformations. It considers complications, the importance of interdisciplinary work, ultrasonography in diagnosis, obstructive uropathies diagnosed in utero with postnatal outcome, and various psychological and ethical problems.

Volume 20

Historical Aspects of Pediatric Surgery

Editor: P. P. Pickham

1986. 119 figures. X, 285 pages. ISBN 3-540-15960-6

Contents: *P. P. Rickham:* Preface. - *W. Ch. Hecker:* The History of Paediatric Surgery in Germany. - *J. Prévot:* The History of Paediatric Surgery in France. - *Th. Ehrenpreis:* 100 Years of Paediatric Surgery in Stockholm, with Personal Memories from the Last 50 Years. - *D. Anagnostopoulos, D. Pellerin:* Cradle of Paediatric Surgery. - *C. A. Montagnani:* Paediatric Surgery in Islamic Medicine from Middle Age to Renaissance. - *A. H. Bill:* William E. Ladd. - *J. Crooks:* Denis Browne: Colleague. - *P. P. Rickham:* Denis Browne: Surgeon. - *II. W. Clatworthy:* Robert E. Gross. - *U. G. Stauffer:* Max Grob. - *P. P. Rickham:* The Dawn of Paediatric Surgery. - *N. A. Myers:* The History of Oesophageal Atresia and Tracheo-Oesophageal Fistula. - *E. Mrozik, T. A. Angerpointner:* Historical Aspects of Hydrocephalus. - *A. F. Schärli:* The History of Colostomy in Childhood. - *D. Cass:* Hirschsprung's Disease: A Historical Review. - *E. H. Strach:* Club-Foot through the Centuries. - *M. Perko:* The History of Treatment of Cleft Lip and Palate. - *J. A. Haller:* Professor Bochdalek and his Hernia - Then and Now. - *R. E. Abdel-Halim:* Paediatric Urology 1000 Years Ago. - *V. A. J. Swain:* Sketches of Surgical Cases drawn in 1884-1887 at The East London Hospital for Children, Shadwell.

Springer-Verlag
Berlin Heidelberg New York
London Paris Tokyo

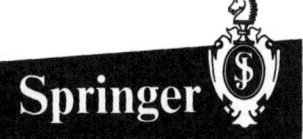

Springer

W. Ch. Hecker

Surgical Correction of Intersexual Genitalia and Female Genital Malformation

With a Section on Pediatric Endocrinology by D. Knorr
Translated from the German by T. C. Telger

1985. 27 figures in 82 separate illustrations. IX, 158 pages
ISBN 3-540-15315-2

This is the first comprehensive, integrated presentation of
the surgical management of intersexual and malformed
female genitalia. It is based on the author's 30 years'
experience in the treatment of such disorders and beauti-
fully illustrated with more than 100 figures prepared
especially for this work.
Since surgical management cannot be treated in isola-
tion, the author includes a discussion of general pathological aspects, pediatric and pediatric-endocrinological
considerations in diagnosis and treatment, and the
psychological ramifications of malformed female genitalia by way of introduction.
The book is designed to provide clear therapeutic para-
meters for all those charged with the care and management of patients suffering from these conditions, be they
pediatric surgeons, pediatricians, urologists, or gynecolo-
gists.

Also available in German

Operative Korrekturen des intersexuellen und des fehlgebildeten weiblichen Genitales

Mit einem kinderendokrinologischen Beitrag von
D. Knorr

Springer-Verlag
Berlin Heidelberg New York
London Paris Tokyo

1985. 27 Abbildungen in 82 Teilabbildungen.
IX, 158 Seiten. ISBN 3-540-15423-X

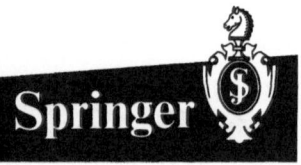
Springer